Committed to the
Insanity and Society in Nineteenth-Century
Quebec and Ontario

Committed to the State Asylum examines the evolution of the asylum as the response to insanity in nineteenth-century Quebec and Ontario. Focusing on the creation and development of government-funded asylums for the insane – among the largest and most important nineteenth-century institutions in both provinces – James Moran argues that asylum development was the result of complex relationships among a wide array of people, including state inspectors and administrators, asylum doctors, local magistrates, jail surgeons, religious authorities, and the relatives and neighbours of those who were considered to be insane.

Unlike other studies, *Committed to the State Asylum* shows the important role that the community played in shaping the asylum and tackles the thorny issue of state development, explaining how state asylums developed differently in each province. Moran considers Canada's pioneering institutional efforts at dealing with the criminally insane and why those efforts lasted only a short time, shedding new light on the debate about the nature and extent of state involvement in nineteenth-century Canadian society.

Committed to the State Asylum offers new insights into the ways in which both ordinary families and the state understood and responded to those they thought had crossed the boundaries of sane behaviour.

JAMES E. MORAN is a Hannah Postdoctoral Fellow at the University of Pennsylvania. He has published articles in *Canadian Bulletin* of *Medical History, History of Psychiatry*, and *Histoire Sociale/ Social History*, and is currently teaching medical history at York University.

MCGILL-QUEEN'S ASSOCIATED MEDICAL SERVICES
(HANNAH INSTITUTE) Studies in the History of Medicine,
Health, and Society
Series Editors: S.O. Freedman and J.T.H. Connor

Volumes in this series have financial support from Associated
Medical Services, Inc., through the Hannah Institute for the
History of Medicine program.

Committed to the State Asylum

Insanity and Society in Nineteenth-Century Quebec and Ontario

JAMES E. MORAN

McGill-Queen's University Press
Montreal & Kingston · London · Ithaca

© McGill-Queen's University Press 2000
ISBN 0-7735-2122-4 (cloth)
ISBN 0-7735-2189-5 (paper)

Legal deposit fourth quarter 2000
Bibliothèque nationale du Québec

Printed in Canada on acid-free paper

This book has been published with the help of a grant
from the Humanities and Social Sciences Federation of
Canada, using funds provided by the Social Sciences
and Humanities Research Council of Canada.

McGill-Queen's University Press acknowledges the
financial support of the Government of Canada through
the Book Publishing Industry Development Program
(BPIDP) for its activities. It also acknowledges the
support of the Canada Council for the Arts for its
publishing program.

Canadian Calatoguing in Publication Data

Moran, James E.
    Committed to the state asylum : insanity and society in
    nineteenth-century Quebec and Ontario
    (McGill-Queen's/Associated Medical Services (Hannah
        Institute) studies in the history of medicine ; 10)
    Includes bibliographical references and index.
    ISBN 0-7735-2122-4 (bnd)
    ISBN 0-7735-2189-5 (pbk)
        1. Psychiatric hospitals–Quebec (Province)–History–19th
    century.   2. Psychiatric hospitals–Ontario–History–19th
    century.   3. Mentally ill–Institutional care–Quebec (Province)–
    History–19th century.   4. Mentally ill–Institutional care–
    Ontario–History–19th century.   I. Title.   II. Series.
    RC447.M67 2001   362.2'1'0971409034   C00-901018-1

This book was typeset by True to Type in 10.5/13 Sabon.

For my parents

Contents

Acknowledgments

This book has benefited from the help of many colleagues over the past seven years. Susan Houston has provided an ideal combination of space for intellectual growth and timely guidance, especially in the writing of the PhD thesis out of which it has emerged. Her enthusiasm for the subject has been a tremendous benefit. I would also like to thank Kate McPherson, Georgina Feldberg, Nicholas Rogers, Wendy Mitchinson, Craig Heron, Paul Antze, and Bettina Bradbury for their helpful criticism at various stages of my work. Lisa-Anne Chilton and Jim Moran have offered tireless assistance in all stages of the manuscript from its conception to its final form. It is a much better work as a result of their efforts. Thomas E. Brown, Jay Cassel, and Geoffrey Reaume have also shaped this book in constructive ways. I am especially grateful to Jean-Marie Fecteau for his encouragement and his willingness to share his knowledge of the records of the provincial secretary related to his work on the "Projet d'incarcération" at the Université de Québec à Montréal. The manuscript reviewers of the Aid to Scholarly Publications Programme and the Hannah Institute for the History of Medicine have helped me reconsider some arguments and clarify and sharpen others. John Zucchi, editor at McGill-Queen's University Press, has been both enthusiastic and helpful throughout the publication process. Jane McWhinney has improved the final text with her invaluable editorial work.

I would like to thank my friend Gerry O'Donnell, whose hospitality in Ottawa afforded me the opportunity to grind out the necessary hours at the National Archives. This book would not have been possible without his generosity and friendship.

At the National Archives of Canada, Pat Kennedy shared with me her expert knowledge on nineteenth-century primary sources. I would also like to thank the helpful staff at the Archives of Ontario, especially archivists Karen Bergsteinsson and Leon Warmski.

This book relies on a range of primary documents that refer to people considered to be insane in the nineteenth century, many of whom became patients in Ontario and Quebec asylums for the insane. The names of these people (and in some cases the names of their families) have been replaced by pseudonyms in this book. However, the files from which information concerning all such cases has been drawn are identified in the notes.

Committed to the State Asylum

Interpreting Sophie's World

By the spring of 1853 Sophie Mercier's behaviour had become alarming to her family and neighbours. Sophie, wife to François Dussault and mother of several children, was about thirty-eight years old and lived in the parish of St Jean Baptiste des Ecureuils in Canada East. Over the previous few months her family and her parish priest had noticed that she was exhibiting an unhealthy obsession with religion, and her husband had come to believe that she posed a physical threat to their children.

The apparent mental breakdown of Sophie Mercier was critical for the whole family. Given the onerous duties of married women in mid-nineteenth-century rural Quebec, which included planting and harvesting the "kitchen" garden, managing the poultry and dairy, baking, cooking, washing, maintaining the household, and rearing the children, Sophie's inability to perform her traditional roles as wife and mother would have exacerbated the hardships of an already difficult way of life. Moreover, the timing of Sophie's troubles near the start of the ploughing season in St Jean Baptiste des Ecureuils would have made it difficult for François to spend much time with her. His need to be absent may in part explain why he resorted to confining Sophie during the day by tying her to the house.

Over the next year and a half the crisis precipitated by Sophie's mental condition became more acute. She tried to drown herself and kill herself with a knife. Neither suicide attempt was successful, but the large unhealed incision on her throat was a lingering visual reminder of her distressed mental state. Her condition began to strain the limits of her husband's tolerance.

But in mid-nineteenth-century Quebec there were few available alternatives to continued management and care of an insane individual within a family. One common strategy was removal of the person to the local jail. A justice of the peace was usually responsible for overseeing this process. The insane person was committed to jail on a charge of being "loose idle and disorderly," or more frequently of being "dangerous to be at large." This practice would effectively remove someone like Sophie from her home into the unpredictable and chaotic environment of a local colonial house of punishment. There she would co-exist with a variety of offenders including petty criminals, debtors, prostitutes, and juvenile offenders. In the local jail her condition might be the object of some medical attention by the physician in charge of the inmates' general health. There she would remain until she was retrieved by her family or friends, or transferred to another institution.

François did not resort to the local jail. He discussed the situation with his parish priest, Father J. Gingras, a local figure of religious and moral authority with some degree of formal education. Through Father Gingras, François petitioned on 31 October to the provincial secretary of Lower Canada for the committal of his wife as a pauper patient to the Beauport Lunatic Asylum near the city of Quebec. Although well-disposed to the petition, the provincial secretary demanded that official supporting documentation be forwarded with the new "patient": a certificate of insanity from a local physician, a completed questionnaire about Sophie's personal history, and a certificate from a local authority testifying to the inability of Sophie's family to contribute to her maintenance at the asylum. Several weeks later, on 11 December, Sophie and her documentation were sent by horse-drawn sleigh to Quebec's first purpose-built asylum for the insane.

As she passed through the gated entrance of the Beauport Lunatic Asylum, Sophie may well have been struck by the imposing architecture of her new residence. Its massive structure was unlike anything in the rural parish of St Jean Baptiste des Ecureuils. Sophie's experience at the asylum would have been as dislocating and alien to her as the institution's architecture. The logic of daily life at the asylum was built loosely around the prevailing paradigm of treatment called "moral therapy," which consisted essentially of closely supervised work, religion, and recreation.

After an initial interview with Beauport's resident physician, new patients were admitted by attendants to the ward appropriate to their sex, their medical diagnosis, and their behaviour. Thereafter, patients were quickly introduced to the daily regimen of asylum life. Officially, the typical asylum day was marked by set periods for eating and sleeping, and a limited range of supervised activities. Sophie would likely have been encouraged to perform duties deemed appropriate to females, which included sewing, mending, knitting, and helping the paid staff with cleaning and cooking. Regular religious services were provided for patients, as were entertainments such as dramatic performances, cards, draughts, and daily excursions within and beyond the asylum grounds, as well as a library for selected reading. She would have had regular contact with ward attendants who were responsible for the daily care of patients and for putting the treatment strategies of the asylum's medical directors into effect. But she would rarely have seen the asylum physician as there were too many patients for regular medical contact. While trying to adjust to this new kind of existence, Sophie would certainly have been affected by the dense crowding of her new environment. She now lived with about three hundred other patients.

As part of her treatment, Sophie might have been given hot or cold baths. If her behaviour became difficult at Beauport, she might also have been confined with a strait-jacket, muffs, or bed straps – or placed in solitary confinement. The incentive to behave well was high. Both male and female wards were organized according to patients' conduct. Had Sophie adapted well to asylum life, she would have found herself moved into the less crowded and less violent atmosphere of the better wards of the asylum. But a patient could be moved in either direction.

Beneath this official institutional regimen organized and directed by the medical directors of the Beauport Asylum, there existed a complicated institutional subculture that confronted new asylum patients such as Sophie. This subculture was created by relationships among patients, and between patients and attendants. It often defied official asylum policy and could be intimidating and even violent. The line between therapy and coercion could be blurred for the overworked and untrained working-class attendants at the asylum. Patients, for their part, had their own ways of resisting the authority of asylum attendants and medical officers. In order to get her allotted share of food and limit the frequency of harassment or even assault, Sophie would have soon had to learn to navigate skilfully through the subculture of asylum life.

It was evident from the start that Sophie did not cope well in her new environment. During her first week at the asylum she refused to eat or drink, and when her husband visited her, he became very concerned by her condition. He also worried about the effect of her departure on the whole family. The loss of the female head of his household, however mentally distressed she may have been, was evidently taking a heavy toll.

Soon after Sophie's committal to the Beauport Asylum, Father Gingras wrote to Father Bolduc, the Catholic chaplain to the asylum. Gingras noted François's strong desire to have her return to her family, and his intention to build a separate room for her in his house for use when her behaviour became unmanageable. Bolduc wrote to the chairman of the Board of Commissioners of the Beauport Asylum, who in turn forwarded the request to the provincial secretary. After eight days in the lunatic asylum, Sophie was sent home.[1]

The complex world of Sophie's social interactions has been subjected to a wide variety of interpretations by historians and other academics. Writers on nineteenth-century insanity have emphasized certain aspects of Sophie's world over others, and have attributed to them a range of contrasting implications.

Until the 1960s academic work on the subject of insanity in the nineteenth century focused on aspects of Sophie's world related to the insane asylum itself and to the physicians and administrators who constructed and revised the new institutional response to insanity that it represented. Although they never dealt specifically with the asylum experience of individuals such as Sophie, the perspective of these early historians was that the asylum was a humanitarian innovation of major therapeutic benefit to its patients. This meliorist, or Whig, approach portrayed the pre-asylum period as a nightmare for the insane. According to this view, although the asylum could be criticized for its administrative shortcomings and even for the primitive nature of its earliest medical tenets, on the whole it ushered in a long period of institutional and professional progress in the diagnosis and treatment of the mentally ill.[2]

With the publication of his *Folie et déraison: histoire de la folie à l'âge classique* in 1961, Foucault stood this meliorist interpretation of the rise of the asylum and of the psychiatric profession on its head. In Foucault's view, far from liberating the insane from a dark history of brutality, and far from establishing the basis for an enlightened institution-based curative psychiatry, the inauguration of the asylum ushered in an era of unprecedented oppression of the mad. With the coming of the asylum, a "gigantic moral imprisonment" displaced a period of relative autonomy and freedom for the insane.[3] For Foucault experiences such as Sophie's in the Beauport Asylum were part of a complex exercise in the social control of the mad.

Foucault's work sparked both controversy[4] and historiographical innovation. In the 1970s David Rothman and Andrew Scull presented soberly critical revisionist accounts of the rise of the asylum.[5] Writing from differing perspectives (Rothman a left-liberal and Scull a neo-marxist), both situated themselves in critical relation to both Foucault's work and to the "march of progress" school of psychiatric history.[6] In Rothman's view, the rise of a range of institutions in the United States, including asylums for the insane, stemmed primarily from a growing lack of confidence in the traditional colonial mechanisms that had assured social cohesion in the antebellum community. The traditional means of dealing with the insanity of individuals like Sophie were no longer considered effective. And, perhaps more important, Sophie's derangement was no longer considered inevitable but rather to result in large measure from "a defect in community organization." According to Rothman, in the early nineteenth century there was a growing sense among reformers that debilitating social ills such as mental alienation could be dealt with and possibly eliminated through the creation of purpose-built institutions: the penitentiary for criminals, the almshouse for the poor, the asylum for the insane. He goes on to argue that despite the early promise held out for such institutions as the asylum, they failed completely in their original aims. Yet, according to Rothman, asylums like the one used to sequester Sophie Mercier did serve a much less humanitarian function as useful locations for the management and custodial treatment of those whom society deemed to be deviant.

Like Rothman, Andrew Scull parted company with the Whig interpretation of Sophie's world, characterizing the nineteenth-century insane asylum as a convenient dumping ground for those unwanted by society. But it was Scull's view that nineteenth-century malaise about existing mechanisms of social cohesion and control centred on tensions caused by major developments in capitalist production. Scull rejected the links made by others between industrialization, urbanization, and the rise of the asylum. In his view, the key factor was the alteration of society by the market economy (starting in mid-eighteenth-century England) which destroyed pre-existing socioeconomic relations between the higher and lower social orders. As the market economy forced more people into waged work for subsistence and simultaneously dissolved the "reciprocal bonds of patronage, deference, and dependence" of the old paternalistic social order, both rural and urban families became unable to bear the burden of care for their insane relatives.[7]

Scull further argued that with the bourgeoisie's rise to prominence during the same period, this powerful class became intolerant of the growing numbers of idle people resorting to poor relief because of poverty brought on by changing and volatile market conditions. The solution to this problem, in the eyes of the bourgeoisie, was to be achieved by institutionalizing unproductive members of the lower orders according to their type of social deviancy. In the case of those considered insane, the state asylum emerged (along with a fledgling psychiatric profession to legitimize it) as the most logical solution. According to Scull, then, the fate of men and women like Sophie was shaped both by the socioeconomic dislocations of the time, which severely compromised the caring capacities of the family, and by the bourgeoisie's endorsement of the state asylum for the containment of one of society's unproductive groups.

The work of Gerald Grob was also important in the literature of asylum history during this period. While distancing himself from a strictly progressive interpretation of institutional development, Grob nevertheless cast a decidedly conservative anchor into a historiography that was becoming more and more critical of the establishment and subsequent development of the asylum.[8] Grob maintained that asylum reformers and psychiatrists had the best of intentions in their creation of a purpose-built institutional response to individuals like Sophie. Several decades into the nineteenth century, however, major social and economic transformations unforeseen by the first generation of asylum builders adversely affected, and eventually derailed, the humanitarian course of the asylum movement.

Industrialization, urban expansion, state policy, and, in the United States, massive influxes of immigrants combined to turn asylums into crowded, ineffective custodial versions of their predecessors.[9]

Despite the sharp differences of opinion between Whig historians, revisionists like Foucault, Rothman, and Scull, and neo-Whig historians like Grob on the significance of the rise and development of the asylum, there are areas of similarity in the ways these writers approached their analyses of the world of nineteenth-century individuals such as Sophie Mercier. First, they all tended to prioritize the same elements from Sophie's world – the asylum, its creators, and its therapeutic philosophy and practice. Second, they all de-emphasized or ignored other components of stories such as Sophie's, especially the circumstances precipitating committal to the asylum, and the personal experiences of asylum patients.

The similarity in the approaches of these historians stemmed in part from their use of the same types of primary sources – government reports and correspondence related to the asylum, reports from asylum psychiatrists, government inquiries, correspondence between asylum and state officials, and the writings of leading theoretical psychiatrists, often referred to in the nineteenth and early twentieth century as alienists. The highly political nature of the debate among these historians paradoxically helps account for the similarities in their approaches. This period of asylum historiography was (and for some still is) characterized above all by fierce disagreement over whether the creation of lunatic asylums was essentially a benevolent process, or whether the undertaking was a more complex and less benevolent project related to a desire for greater social control.[10]

A deluge of more recent works on nineteenth-century asylum and psychiatric history are, on the whole, less theoretically driven and more analytically open-ended than those of the first wave of revisionist writers.[11] Through the use of a variety of methodological approaches and the exploration of an increasingly broad range of primary sources (including patient records, documents pertaining to asylum committal and discharge, and correspondence between the asylum and the families of the insane), this growing body of literature has opened up the field dramatically.

Most of these recent accounts explored previously uncharted archival territory in the history of insanity, the asylum, and the families of the insane. In these works, situations such as Sophie's became much more difficult to theorize at a macro-historical level.

For this wave of writers, it was important to recreate a patient's experience in the asylum and to consider more thoroughly the events leading to an individual's committal. Partly because these historians focused on specific asylums and more minute subjects of historical inquiry, the world of the psychiatric patient became seemingly more complex and appeared to defy explanation through the exclusive application of one body of theory.

In a recent historiographical article, Thomas E. Brown has argued that the large corpus of asylum history studies produced in the 1980s and early 1990s can be characterized chiefly by its retreat from theory and "the political." Brown contends that two interrelated factors explain asylum historians' recent disinclination to set their studies within a more ambitious theoretical context. First, the fierce historiographical debate among revisionists and between Whigs and revisionists in the late 1970s and the 1980s was seen by subsequent historians to have stagnated in a pitched rhetorical battle over the concept of "social control." Partly in their efforts to distance themselves from the increasing stigma of the social-control label, subsequent historians retreated from a thorough theoretical consideration of their topic.

Brown's second point is that recent scholars of the history of psychiatry were influenced by selective components of the "new social history." They embarked upon ambitious archival projects that focused on micro-historical subjects (usually the history of a single insane asylum) in an effort to "rescue" asylum workers, patients, and the relatives of the insane from the "condescension of posterity"[12] and build an empirical base upon which to create a new interpretation of the history of madness and the asylum. But, according to Brown, this direction was taken without addressing the complicated neo-marxist and post-structuralist theoretical debates informing similar history in other fields. In Brown's view, these works constitute a "neo-revisionist" perspective which, although rich in archival research, is averse to overarching political or theoretical considerations.[13]

Brown's article is a clarion call to prospective writers on the history of insanity and psychiatry not to ignore the theoretical and historiographical contributions of their revisionist predecessors.[14] He notes that although revisionists disagreed with each other they all agreed on the importance of the relationship between responses to insanity and the wider social, economic, and political contexts of the societies from which they emerged.

Since the publication of Brown's overview of historiography, there is evidence to suggest that the history of asylum studies is coming full circle. Rejecting the revisionist interpretations of Scull, Rothman, Foucault, and others, Peter Keating argues that moral therapy is best regarded as "a new breakthrough in the domain of medical thought."[15] Even more striking in its curt denunciation of the full range of revisionist writers is Edward Shorter's recent account of the history of psychiatry from the pre-asylum era to the present.[16] With Shorter we are back to a meliorist interpretation of the history of psychiatry, which sees the recent "biological approach to psychiatry – treating mental illness as a genetically influenced disorder of brain chemistry – [as] a smashing success." In this account the historical legitimacy of past psychiatric endeavour is measured against the present reality (in Shorter's view) of mental illness as a biologically determined disorder.[17] Also notable in the work of Shorter and Keating is a lack of interest in the primary sources and methodologies explored by the social historians of psychiatry of the 1980s and 1990s. Both authors construct an account of Sophie's world in which perceptions and responses of asylum patients, workers, and community are again relegated to the shadows of marginal significance.

While a revival of meliorist accounts marks one identifiable trend in recent histories of psychiatry and the asylum, historian David Wright suggests that a constellation of other studies points historiography in still another direction.[18] According to Wright, the weight of historical evidence in several social histories of the asylum throws into question many previously held assumptions about the nature of the nineteenth-century asylum. Wright argues that recent examinations of the motives and circumstances prompting households and local communities to commit patients to asylum care reorients the historian away from the primacy of the psychiatric profession in asylum development towards the centrality of the family in asylum committal. These studies also implicitly question the extent to which asylum development "medicalized" attitudes about insanity at the local level in the nineteenth century. In Wright's view, "the confinement of the insane" is best considered "as a pragmatic response of households to the stresses of industrialization."[19] From this perspective, the circumstances that led Sophie's family and community to commit her to the asylum are considered not only to be important but perhaps to be the driving forces shaping the process of asylum development.[20]

Where does this book stand in relation to a field marked by such rapidly shifting and overlapping interpretations? In general terms, it combines an appreciation of the contributions made by the first wave of revisionist writers with a respect for the methodological and analytical innovations of the new social historians of insanity and the asylum. It addresses the call of historiographers such as Thomas Brown for a more contextualized history of the asylum. It also shares with the work of David Wright and others the opinion that the study of the process of patient committal is crucial to a reconceptualization of the history of the asylum and insanity. To the extent that the historian can uncover it, Sophie's story as a whole is thus relevant, with all its potential analytical and theoretical implications.[21]

This study traces the social history of the lunatic asylum in Ontario and Quebec in the course of the nineteenth century. As a model for the management and treatment of insanity, the asylum ideal was already an intellectual force to be reckoned with in the United States, England and elsewhere by the time either province decided to adopt such institutions. Thus asylum advocates in Quebec and Ontario were drawing upon models already developed and accepted. Nevertheless, asylum development in each province was affected by a complex synthesis of pressures generated by the conflicting interactions of people from a hierarchy of social and economic circumstances – government inspector, asylum superintendent, local legal or religious authority, jail surgeon, and relatives or neighbours of the person considered to be insane.

These formative interactions were played out in a society in which power was unequally distributed. Government officials, asylum advocates, and medical administrators exercised considerable power and authority over families who decided to commit a relative to the asylum and over the "insane" individuals themselves as they underwent the process of becoming asylum patients. This situation was, of course, consistent with the prevailing social structure of nineteenth-century Canada. In many respects, the unevenness of power embodied in these heirarchical social relationships accounted for the patterns of asylum development unique to Ontario and Quebec. But this socioeconomic reality did not prevent groups with less power from making their mark in shaping the nineteenth-century asylum.

1 Manipulating a Monopoly: The State and the "Farming-Out System" in Quebec

A form of institutional care and treatment of the insane developed in nineteenth-century Quebec that was known by its contemporaries as the "farming-out" system. The farming-out system resulted from the interactions of the provincial state, with its concerns about the costs of asylum provision, and a group of Quebec physicians, driven by professional and proprietary ambitions. The farming-out arrangements reached between the state and these physicians, the proprietors of Quebec's first permanent lunatic asylum at Beauport, were quickly consolidated into a monopoly in the asylum care of the insane.

Once established, this state-sanctioned medical monopoly became firmly entrenched in Quebec. Its creation and growth led to a relationship between insanity and the state that contrasted markedly with the system that developed in Ontario. The Quebec model can best be understood by examining certain patterns of development that stemmed from Beauport's long-standing monopoly status.

The contractual negotiations between the proprietors of the Beauport Lunatic Asylum and the state reveal that this monopoly became stronger during the middle decades of the nineteenth century. This concentration of power had much to do with the managerial prowess and ambition of the asylum proprietors. As the scope and scale of care at the Beauport Lunatic Asylum grew, so too did its proprietors' ability to negotiate more favourable terms from the state during each contract renewal and between contracts. Negotiations were not completely one-sided, however. The state did succeed in becoming more intrusive in the affairs of the asylum over the course of the century. But on the whole the proprietors wielded enormous power in the development of their institution at Beauport.

The grip of this medical monopoly becomes particularly evident when one examines the extent to which the asylum owners were able to limit state inspection and supervision of asylum affairs. The Board of Commissioners of the Beauport Asylum got along reasonably well with the asylum owners because the board endorsed almost every measure the proprietors took. Although the board frequently voiced concerns about overcrowding at the asylum, the circumstances leading to crises in patient population were always too complex to allow the commissioners to lay blame solely on the proprietors. Even the creation in 1859 of the Board of Inspectors of Prisons, Asylums and Public Charities for the United Province of Canada East and West failed to substantially reduce the authority of the Beauport medical proprietors over the institutional care of the insane.

Not only did the Beauport proprietors' protection of their monopoly curtail state inspection; it also limited the extent of asylum expansion elsewhere in the province. When a state-controlled lunatic asylum was eventually established at St Jean in 1861, it was by all accounts a very small and unsuccessful counterpart to Beauport. Criticized by asylum inspectors and the the Beauport proprietors for being grossly inadequate to the needs of the insane, the St Jean Provincial Lunatic Asylum became a foil against which the Beauport Lunatic Asylum was favourably compared. This comparison in effect augmented the power and status of the proprietary institution. St Jean was a relatively brief and unsuccessful experiment in state-run asylum care that did little to alter the Beauport monopoly.

In a more successful attempt to break the monopoly status of the Beauport Asylum, the state negotiated major asylum contracts with the Sisters of Providence. This Catholic order and its representatives, however, resisted government interference with the management and organization of their asylums as fiercely as the Beauport proprietors did. It was not until after the 1887 Royal Commission

Table 1   Système des Loges (Number of Loges and Their Location)

City	Date	Loges
Quebec	1720	6
	1802	12
	1820s	6
Montreal	1802	8
Trois-Rivières	1808	6
Total	—	38

Source: Table compiled from information found in André Cellard, *Histoire de la folie au Québec de 1600 à 1850* (Montréal: 1991)

on Lunatic Asylums in the Province of Quebec, which investigated the impasse between the asylum proprietors and the provincial government, that the state was finally able to exercise any real degree of control over the institutional organization and regulation of insanity. This royal commission, its recommendations, and the state's subsequent actions highlighted the unique relationship between insanity and the state that had developed in Quebec by the end of the nineteenth century.

In the early nineteenth century, state involvement in the institutional management of the insane in Lower Canada had taken the form of a *système des loges* run by the religious orders of the general hospitals in Montreal, Quebec, and Three Rivers. (See Table 1.) Each *loge* had room for one patient. As early as 1720, six *loges* had been built at the Quebec General Hospital for the insane, supported financially by contract with the colonial government. In 1801 a law was passed to perpetuate this arrangement, giving the religious orders at Montreal, Quebec, and Three Rivers up to £1,000 per year to care for the insane and for abandoned children. A Commission for Insane Persons and Foundlings was established to take responsibility for admissions. The commissioners soon found this grant insufficient to provide for upkeep of the cells, medical and non-medical care, and food and provisions for the insane, and they frequently petitioned for increases in funds beyond the original government grant.[1] This state-sponsored system of management was increasingly perceived to be unacceptable by commissioners, other prominent citizens, and government officials.[2] Critical assessment of the *système des loges* was especially evident from about 1816 until the establishment of the Beauport Lunatic Asylum in 1845. Opposition focused both on the inhumane conditions of the *loges*, and on the impossibility of curing the insane under that system of care. In a report to Governor Sherbrooke, Commissioner Dr W. Hackett claimed that the hospital cells worked completely "against the principles that might give hope for healing the insane."[3] A typical grand jury presentment described "the misery" of the insane lodged in the Montreal General Hospital as "extreme."[4]

By 1824 criticism of the state-funded *système des loges* was accompanied by calls for the establishment of a permanent, publicly-funded lunatic asylum.[5] In 1825, after "painful" inspection, Lieutenant Governor Francis Burton described conditions in the cells for the insane in Quebec and Montreal:

[They are] merely places of confinement, to prevent the inmates from injuring themselves and others, but [they] do not admit of those arrangements for cure, or proved and benevolent mode of treatment prescribed. Defective, however, as those places are, yet they are so inadequate to the wants of the Community, that the Gaols are not only resorted to, for the confinement of persons convicted of insanity, but of several poor and dangerous Lunatics, to the great annoyance of Prisoners, impediment to classification and impossibility of affording relief to those unhappy persons themselves. A total change of system, with a concentration of means and conveniences, can alone produce that improvement so much to be wished for.[6]

The Lieutenant Governor recommended that the Assembly make "adequate provision for building and furnishing a Lunatic Asylum for the whole Province, with sufficient airing grounds, in a proper situation for bodily health, medical assistance, and regular superintendence, whereby to promote the cure or mitigation of that most melancholy of human maladies." Burton's recommendations led to the formation of a special committee, which, although agreeing whole-heartedly with the findings of the Lieutenant Governor, nevertheless regretted that the "situation of the funds of the province" did not allow for the adoption of the plan.[7]

As Burton's account indicates, beyond the question of therapeutic efficacy, dissatisfaction with the *système des loges* also stemmed from the fact that the hospitals' small patient capacity made it necessary to house the insane also in district jails. The resulting mix of different forms of social deviancy in local prisons was considered more and more unacceptable in Canada (as in England and the United States) over the course of the nineteenth century. Although never practised to any great extent in the first part of the century, the ideology of separating and classifying the "problem" groups in society for specialized institutional confinement was frequently voiced in Lower and Upper Canada.[8] The insane were considered particularly in need of sequestering from the mass of prison inmates because of their unusual and highly disruptive behaviour.

The problem of the insane in the prison population of Lower Canada was intensified in 1831 when the Grey Nuns at the Montreal Hôtel Dieu refused to take any more insane persons into their loges.[9] The Montreal Jail thus became the only institution for the insane of that district. In 1837 this situation led Lieutenant Governor Sir John Colbourne to call for a committee mandated to establish a temporary asylum for the relief of the insane and to purchase a property in the Montreal district that would serve as the future site for a permanent asylum.[10] Perhaps due to the outbreak of the rebellions, appointments to this committee were not officially made until 29 March 1839.[11]

Further support for the establishment of state institutions for the insane was voiced at the imperial level in the Durham Report, published on 11 February 1839, following the rebellions. Information on the state of care for the insane was provided to Durham by Sir John Doratt, MD, who deployed a combination of medical, economic, and moral arguments to back his call for the opening of public lunatic asylums in the districts of Quebec and Montreal. In his "Observations on the Custody of the Insane and the Expediency of a Public Lunatic Asylum," Doratt reiterated by-then familiar descriptions of the therapeutic inefficacies and deplorable conditions of the *système des loges*. He also noted "the disgraceful system of incarcerating the insane in the common gaol with the culprit and prisoners committed for every offence." In advocating the establishment of state lunatic asylums in the Lower Province, Doratt relied heavily on the English and European medical professions' claims to expertise in the management and cure of insanity. Referring to the cells of the General Hospitals and the local prisons he noted:

It is a fact well ascertained that insane persons held in close confinement, and thereby prevented from receiving the natural and requisite effects of fresh air, and likewise deprived of the means to exercise the body, are by such deprivations exposed to the fearful effects of the lower decomposed blood and arrested circulation, from which not infrequently mortification of the lower extremities is the result; and if the cerebral structure of an insane person should be pressed upon from any irregularity of venal circulation, the disease of insanity will in all probability be much aggravated.

Doratt wished to replace this medically dangerous form of management with the therapeutic approach of the insane asylum based on "the united talent of several medical men, who, having devoted their time and abilities to the subject, and by their labours having acquired extensive knowledge thereon, have given to the world a mass of information consolidated into facts founded upon numerous and extended experiments."[12]

The insane asylum was preferable not only on scientific medical grounds. According to Doratt, it was also a fiscally superior alternative to the "enormous expenses incurred by the legislature of Lower Canada for the maintenance in solitary confinement of a few insane poor in the [districts] of Quebec and of Montreal." The consolidation of the insane from the various *loges* and district jails into purpose-built curative asylums for the insane would give the legislature a better return for the money which it allocated for that purpose.

The final component to Doratt's argument focused on the moral imperatives of lunatic asylum care. He, in company with scores of reformers of his day, considered the asylum to be more humane than any form of treatment that was then provided either by other institutions or within the family or community setting. Through the application of "moral management," Doratt claimed, at least 50 or 60 per cent of the insane could be cured and restored to their families and communities.[13] It was his view that the presence of the insane scattered about in Lower Canada produced "the worst influence over the moral character of society at large, particularly in the more populous districts, inhabited principally by Canadians."[14]

This latter statement can be interpreted in more than one way. Asylum promoters felt that the presence of the insane in the community was disruptive and unhealthy for both patient and family, and they almost always recommended the patient's prompt removal from the social milieu of "morbid associations" to the curative influence of the asylum setting.[15] According to André Cellard and Dominique Nadon, however, Doratt's statement becomes much more significant when it is considered in the context of post-rebellion Durhamite Lower Canada. In their view, Dorrat "went so far as to make a connection between the Rebellions and the existence of lunatics at large among the French-Canadians." This is perhaps too literal a reading of Doratt. However, there is no doubt that the Durham project to re-establish social order in the post-rebellion Canadas was in large measure to be effected, in theory at least, through the establishment of such "progressive" British institutions as schools, prisons, penitentiaries and lunatic asylums.[16]

In the case of the lunatic asylum, the Durham Report resulted in an initial flurry of activity in Lower Canada. On 29 March 1839 the committee that John Colbourne had called for two years earlier took formal shape with the appointment of nine members. The committee wasted no time in selecting and purchasing an appropriate site for a permanent asylum on the Côte Saint-Antoine in the district of Montreal. Pending the construction of the permanent asylum, the commissioners set out to find temporary relief for the insane, eventually opting to set up a provisional asylum on the third floor of the Montreal district jail on 1 November 1839.

The temporary lunatic asylum in the Montreal district jail remained open much longer than originally intended. In fact, after the opening of the provisional lunatic asylum, the provision of a permanent, purpose-built institution remained a low state priority until 1845, when the Beauport Lunatic Asylum was founded. Cellard suggests that the successful repression of the rebellions decreased the sense of urgency to restore order by establishing a permanent lunatic asylum.[17]

The rebellions did indeed precipitate a brief intensification of activity in regard to the establishment of a permanent lunatic asylum. Moreover, as many have pointed out elsewhere, the theory behind permanent asylum provision based on moral therapeutic principles was in many respects in keeping with the perceived need for social control. However, the movement to establish permanent asylum care had begun well before the rebellions in Quebec and carried on in much the same way after them. In the end, despite briefly sparking an increased interest in asylums, it was not the rebellions that ultimately hastened the achievement of a permanent state asylum. It was rather, in Quebec as elsewhere, prolonged lobbying on the part of reformers, and a gradual change in perceptions of the state's responsibility towards, and relationship with, the insane. From an imperial perspective, there was no great urgency to work towards Durham's more abstract and refined vision of the liberal state in the mid-century colonial setting of Lower and Upper Canada. Military and, later, police repression, as well as legal and legislative coercion, were quite sufficient to deal with the immediate concerns of colonial revolt.[18]

Discontent with the existing state of provision for the insane was hardly abated by the establishment of the temporary asylum in the Montreal Jail. Although it differed in scale and in internal organization and management from the *système des loges* of the general hospitals run by the religious orders in Montreal, Quebec, and Three Rivers, petitions and Grand Jury presentments emphasized that the Montreal Jail was both architecturally and therapeutically inadequate to meet the growing population of insane persons in the lower province.[19]

In 1843 Dorothea Dix, the leading asylum advocate in the United States, joined in the call for state provision for the insane in Quebec and Ontario. In a "memorial" to the Legislature of Canada East and West, Dix combined humanitarianism, science, and economics in her endorsement of a "hospital for the insane" in Quebec that would be capable of accommodating from 200 to 250 patients. She recommended provision for incurable lunatics on humanitarian grounds, and a combination of "nursing" and "skilful treatment" for those "whose cases afford hope of recovery." In her typical fashion, Dix was careful not to blame authorities for failing to provide such treatment, but said she felt confident that "humanity" and "good sense" would prevail in future efforts to legislate proper asylum provision. As in her struggles to establish state structures for asylum provision in the United States, Dix carefully linked humanitarian concerns for the plight of the insane with an economic argument: "The accumulation of large numbers of hopeless cases in your prisons ... affords evidence that the longer a proper provision is delayed in your country, the greater are your annual expenses, and these will be found rising year by year, while the application of remedies to existing evils is delayed." By curing insanity, Dix argued, asylums in the long run saved money.[20]

Continuous pressure from a variety of sources for government attention to the plight of the insane eventually led to a more determined response on the part of the state. On 19 August 1844 Governor Metcalfe made it known that the lower province was finally provided with the "opportunity" to "obtain the object desired, that is the proper care of insane persons, with a view to their cure; and also for the attainment of this object at less cost than would be incurred in any other mode."[21] Metcalfe had succinctly captured the colonial state's perception of its role in the care of the insane. In the final analysis, the state required that the humanitarian, professional, and medical arguments of asylum advocates be harmonized with the fiscal concerns of the colonial government if asylum treatment was to be fully endorsed as a state priority.

Metcalfe had received a proposal from two Montreal physicians, Drs Badgely and Sutherland, "to establish an institution for the care and cure of insanes in a salubrious position" in the district of Montreal. The doctors wanted 14 or 15 shillings per week for each patient received. In the proposed arrangement, the government would pay the physicians for the provision and care of patients, while the asylum buildings and grounds would remain the property of the physicians themselves. Metcalfe was pleased with this proposal. Although the existing government expenditure for each insane person was 14 shillings per week in the temporary asylum in Montreal and 11 shillings, 8 pence per week in the Quebec district, the governor was confident that the slightly lower cost currently paid by the state did not include all the charges contained in the estimate given by Badgely and Sutherland.[22] Metcalfe requested that a committee of the Executive Council report on "the expediency and practicability" of the proposal suggested by Badgely and Sutherland and evaluate "the terms ... best calculated to ensure the due care of the patients with the least charge to the Province."[23]

By the time the Executive Council had formed an initial response to the governor's request, two more proposals in addition to that of Badgely and Sutherland were being seriously considered by the colonial government: one from Dr Henry Mount of Montreal, and one from Drs Douglas, Frémont, and Morrin of Quebec City. The Executive Council suggested that all three proposals should be considered on a trial basis for one or two years, and then "permanently adopted after some time of successful experience, or abandoned if found not to answer." But the Executive Council also advised that a final decision on each proposal should be put off until more details on each offer could be obtained.[24]

In response to the government's subsequent call for more detailed proposals, Badgely and Sutherland reported in November 1844 that their asylum would be ready to accept forty-five patients within one month of receiving the sanction of the state. They further assured the provincial secretary that by September of the next year the number of patients could be increased to 175. There was an "abundance of grounds" surrounding the asylum for "bodily exercise and mental recreation" of the insane. The location of the asylum itself was "healthy, elevated, easily accessible and yet perfectly isolated." Their charge of 15 shillings per week per patient was, in their opinion, considerably lower than that levied either in the United States or in Britain for similar accommodation. For such a reasonable rate, the would-be medical proprietors insisted on a contract with the government for a period of no less than ten years.[25]

The second of the three proposals for contracted care of the insane came from Dr Henry Mount. Mount had originally considered converting his "spacious mansion" at Point Claire near Montreal into an asylum for "a limited number of upper or better classes of society who are at present transferred to foreign institutions to the disadvantage of this country." But upon inquiry, he found that there were too few of these cases to warrant a large expenditure for the fitting-out of an asylum. He therefore proposed to the government that he convert his mansion and 30-acre property into an asylum for both private and government patients. In greater detail than the Badgely and Sutherland submission, Mount described his proposed asylum as similar in design and function to those of "Europe or America." It would be based on then-popular moral and medical forms of treatment, with due attention to ventilation, heating, recreation, work, attendant supervision, and the basics of board, lodging, clothing, and washing. Mount also expressed his receptivity to the idea of a government inspectorate of asylum commissioners whose periodic recommendations "in relation to the internal economy of the asylum" he would receive with "deference and attention." Mount would not consider a contract with the government for less than twenty-one years.[26]

The final proposal considered by the government was that of Drs James Douglas, Charles Frémont, and Joseph Morrin of Quebec. In much the same manner as the other two proposals had done, these physicians offered to accommodate forty patients within one month of striking a contract with the government and as many more patients as was necessary after a further period of one year of preparations. Douglas, Frémont, and Morrin argued that the government-owned "Domain Farm" at Beauport near the city of Quebec was the best possible site for the establishment of an asylum for the Quebec district. They asked for 15 shillings per week (or £39 per year) from the government for each patient, and requested a contract for an initial period of three years.[27]

For a variety of reasons, none of these three proposals met with the immediate approval of the state. First, the duration of the contracts proposed by Mount, and by Badgely and Sutherland was considered too long. The government wanted more flexibility to end the relationship with the prospective asylum entrepreneurs in the event that either contract did not work out. Second, it was the view of the governor general that the charge per patient in both proposals was still too high. Rather than accept either of the Montreal district proposals, the Executive Council authorized the commissioners of the temporary lunatic asylum in Montreal to "provide without delay, a suitable place of residence in order that the lunatics may, with the greatest speed, be removed from the Gaol."[28] To the proposal of Drs Douglas, Frémont, and Morrin, the government responded that it opposed the idea of using the Domain Farm as a site for an asylum. Nevertheless, whereas the Montreal district proposals had been rejected outright, the provincial secretary asked the three Quebec physicians for the terms under which they would receive patients from the districts of Quebec and Three Rivers "in the event of [their] providing other suitable premises and accommodation at [their] own cost" for the reception of the insane.[29]

At this stage the government's strategy was beginning to take shape. Uneasy with the proposals from the Montreal area, it hoped that the commissioners of the temporary lunatic asylum could find less expensive accommodation for the insane of that district. For the districts of Quebec and Three Rivers, the government would see if it could not force a better deal with Douglas, Frémont, and Morrin. Consistent with state policy, low-cost accommodation was the priority behind which all other virtues of permanent asylum care were to be aligned.

Financial concerns dominated subsequent negotiations with Douglas, Frémont, and Morrin. The physicians proposed the establishment of an asylum "with extensive grounds for air and exercise, ... good and sufficient food and clothing and attendance, with medical services" at the Manor House at Beauport. This manor, owned by Colonel Gugys, was situated on a 100-acre plot of land. In this proposal, the physicians raised their required fee for each patient from £39 to £45 per year. The physicians argued that the higher fees were initially necessary to offset the costs of establishing the asylum. Should the arrangement with the government be made permanent, the physicians asserted, they would be happy to consider a reduction in fees after two or three years. The government's response to this proposal was to push harder for a lower fee per patient in exchange for a guaranteed three-year contract. But Douglas, Frémont, and Morrin had made their final offer. They rejected any further reduction in patient charges. Finally, on 18 June 1845, the governor general ratified the Executive Council's decision to approve the Quebec physicians' proposal, which by then included the reception of insane persons from the district of St Francis, in addition to those from Quebec and Three Rivers.[30]

Having settled on arrangements for the management of the insane in the eastern part of the province, the government once more turned its attention to the Montreal district. The commissioners of the Montreal Temporary Lunatic Asylum who had been instructed to find a more suitable "house" for the accommodation of the insane had been unsuccessful in their search. Dr Trestler, secretary to the temporary asylum, therefore strongly recommended that the government consider establishing a permanent lunatic asylum on the property originally purchased by the state for that purpose in 1839. He suggested that a system of taxation could be implemented in order to finance the plan.[31]

Not wanting to incur the costs of a state-built asylum, the government rejected Trestler's recommendation and instead reopened communications with Badgely and Sutherland. The government offered to accept the physicians' original offer, but for a limited three-year trial period rather than for the ten years originally proposed. This was essentially the same contract that had been arranged with Douglas, Frémont and Morrin. But Badgely and

Sutherland were unwilling to accept the counter-offer. In their view: "The period of 10 years originally contemplated by us was one which on calculation we found would, if not remunerate, at least guard us from loss; on this modified proposition we have ascertained that no capitalist could be induced to enter upon a venture, the success of which necessarily depends on the time during which he might receive interest on his investment." Adamant that a ten-year contract was essential to safeguard their investment in the management of the insane, the two medical entrepreneurs refused to accept the government's terms.[32]

On 18 July, seven days after Badgely and Sutherland had declined the government's final offer, the provincial secretary received word from James Douglas that he and his partners could provide accommodation for the insane then held at the Montreal Temporary Asylum. Dr Frémont travelled to Montreal to speak personally with the provincial secretary on the matter, suggesting that the asylum could be ready to receive patients from the Montreal Jail by 1 September. On 4 August the government pushed for an earlier reception date and the Quebec physicians acceded, agreeing to advance their opening date to 16 August. Continuing reports from the commissioners of the Montreal Temporary Lunatic Asylum and the warden of the Montreal Jail on the deterioration of their provision for the insane,[33] in conjunction with Badgely and Sutherland's refusal of the government's counter-offer, led the Executive Council to an impasse: "No other alternative is left to [the Governor General] but to accept the proposition" of the three Quebec physicians.[34] By 12 August 1845, Douglas, Frémont, and Morrin had undertaken a three-year contract with the state to accommodate the insane from the districts of Montreal, Quebec, Three Rivers, and St Francis in their Beauport Lunatic Asylum. By 5 October, nineteen patients under the care of the Sisters of the Quebec General Hospital, fifty-two patients from the temporary lunatic asylum in the Montreal Jail, and seven patients under the charge of the Sisters of the General Hospital at Three Rivers were transferred to Beauport. The conclusion of these arrangements marked the beginning of a medical monopoly in the institutional management and care of the insane in Quebec.

Shortly after the establishment of Beauport's monopoly, it became apparent that the government grant allocated to provide for patients at that institution was insufficient to meet growing demand for admissions. By the fall of 1848, the Quebec and Montreal district jails reported that they were accommodating insane inmates because there was no money to commit them to Beauport.[35] In response to their pressure to find accommodation, Dr Trestler (ex-secretary of the temporary lunatic asylum at Montreal) again proposed the creation of an asylum in Montreal on similar terms with the government to those established for the Beauport Asylum. This, Trestler argued, would eliminate the expense and difficulty of transporting the insane from the Montreal district to Beauport.[36] But the colonial government concluded that the expense of setting up an additional institution for the insane would be greater than that of maintaining an enlarged Beauport Asylum, even with the costs of patient transportation taken into account. The executive committee thus recommended a strategy for increasing the number of patients at Beauport. They would bargain with the Beauport proprietors for a reduced fee per patient in the upcoming contract renewal in the fall of 1848.[37]

Both the government and the Beauport Asylum proprietors agreed that the original fee per patient was based on "the short [three-year] period for which the arrangement was made, and on the great and immediate outlay [that was necessary] for fitting up and providing an establishment with furniture, bedding, clothing, &c."[38] A reduction in fees was thus acceptable to both parties. But there was disagreement over how much lower the price per patient would be. Douglas, Frémont, and Morrin proposed a fee schedule set at 15 shillings per week for two-thirds of the patient population, and 10 shillings per week for the remaining one-third. The rationale behind this "sliding scale" was that two-thirds of Beauport's patient population "required constant watchfulness, care, and medical and moral treatment" while the remaining one-third required no curative attention, "being either idiotic from birth, or imbecilic from long continued disease of the brain."[39] The proprietors noted that these reduced fees would permit an additional seventeen patients to the asylum without any additional outlay. But the government considered this reduction insufficient and counter-proposed its own weekly fee structure of 12 shillings and 6 pence for the two-thirds of the patient population "requiring curative treatment," and 10 shillings for the remaining patients.[40] On the basis of these fees, the government was willing to sign a new five-year contract.

Douglas, Frémont, and Morrin grudgingly accepted the reduced fees proposed by the state but requested that the contract be renewed for seven rather than five years. This, they argued, would enable them to construct a new building to separate the curable and incurable patients. A guaranteed seven-year contract was necessary to compensate them for the "considerable expense in the erection and fitting up" of the new building. Under these conditions the asylum proprietors were willing to take in an additional forty-five patients without any further government outlay. The government agreed to the extension, and the renewed contract was signed for the seven-year period from 1 October 1848 to 1 October 1855.[41]

This first contract renewal, relatively simple in its conditions and stipulations, reflected the concerns of both the state and the asylum proprietors. Having found a relatively successful and reliable solution to the problem of provision for the insane, the state wished to perpetuate the arrangement, but wanted a greater number of government patients accommodated at a reduced cost. Here the state was responding to pressure from grand jury presentments and jail reports (especially from Montreal and Quebec) urging the removal of those considered insane from the local prisons to a "proper" place of treatment and management. For their part, the proprietors recognised that a lower fee schedule could be absorbed if they could be guaranteed a sufficiently long contract and a large enough patient allocation to ensure a good return on their investment. An extended contract would enable the asylum owners to expand the asylum and purchase provisions for the insane on more favourable terms, thus in the long run minimizing their expenditure per patient.

In what would become a crucial type of clause in all contracts between the state and the asylum proprietors, the government agreed to commit its complete annual grant for the relief of the insane to send patients to Beauport. It could not contract with any other institution, unless the legislature increased its annual grant for the relief of the insane above £7,500.[42] This clause, energetically fought for by Douglas, Frémont, and Morrin guaranteed Beauport's monopoly status in the face of countless proposals for the establishment of other asylums in the province.

Within a month of signing the new contract, the Beauport proprietors had purchased a new 70-acre property at La Canardière, upon which they planned to build a new, expanded and improved asylum complex. Before beginning construction, they notified the government, explaining that they anticipated that the new asylum would "demand very considerable outlay." They inquired whether it was probable that accommodation might "some time ... be required for a greater number of patients from the different districts, than was contemplated at the time the present arrangement was made as [they] could now at comparatively little additional expense make the necessary provisions for an increased number."[43] Although the government refused to guarantee any increase in Beauport's patient population, the proprietors went ahead with an ambitious construction program, building an asylum that included a large central building with two wings, and a patient capacity of 200, as well as sleeping quarters for an additional 120 patients in the attic of the central building.[44] Despite the lack of a guarantee, the proprietors were banking on a higher demand for their services in the near future.

The proprietors' aggressive expansion strategy placed them in an advantageous position when renegotiating with the state towards the end of their seven-year contract. On 24 November 1853, Douglas, Frémont, and Morrin set forth a much more demanding list of conditions under which they were willing to renew their contract for the care and management of the insane at Beauport. They wanted the next contract to extend for a period of ten years and requested an agreement that "no arrangement will be entered into by government with other parties, until the number of patients under [the proprietors' charge] shall average 250." Moreover, in such an eventuality, the Beauport proprietors wanted to be given an opportunity to erect other buildings to house the surplus patients before the state would consider contracting with other potential proprietors. In the event of the proprietors' willingness to expand provision for an asylum population beyond 250 patients, they wanted the "ceiling" beyond which the state could look elsewhere for accommodation to be set at 300 patients. Douglas, Frémont, and Morrin further requested a clause in the new contract enabling them to claim compensation for loss "should the price of provisions, labour, [and] fuel [rise in the future] higher than at the present time, whether in consequence of war or any other cause." Under these conditions, the proprietors were willing to continue their management and care of the insane in Quebec for the same fees per patient as agreed to under the old contract. They also promised to build a separate institution for "incurable lunatics" to effect better classification and separation of the insane.[45]

In a report endorsing the proprietors' demands, the provincial secretary noted that to date the Beauport Lunatic Asylum had been run by Douglas, Frémont, and Morrin with excellent results, on the most liberal and most advanced principles. Moreover, the Beauport Asylum, as a privately run institution, had not encountered any of the "contentions and innumerable difficulties that institutions such as the Quebec Marine and Emigrant Hospital in Quebec, or the Toronto Provincial Asylum in Ontario, under government control, had experienced." The provincial secretary further commented that the cost of patient care at the Beauport Asylum was lower than at any institution in the United States, and that it also compared favourably with the cost per patient at the Toronto Provincial Asylum, when the expenses incurred by the Beauport proprietors in the construction and improvement of their asylum were taken into account.[46] Thanks to this favourable review, all of the conditions set out by the Beauport proprietors were met in the new contract, which was to extend from 1 October 1855 to 1 October 1865.

But this ten-year contract negotiated between the state and the Beauport proprietors was short-lived. Just over a year after it was signed, Douglas, Frémont, and Morrin petitioned the government, arguing that "pecuniary loss" was the inevitable result of the continuation of the contract under existing conditions. The proprietors insisted that either the fee per patient be increased in a renewed contract to 13 shillings and 9 pence per week for all patients regardless of their medical designation or the state take over responsibility for the asylum by buying out the owners. The government sanctioned the increased fee per patient at the Beauport Asylum, but in return, required that a new limit for accommodation be set at 400 patients. In addition, the clause in the old contract insuring the proprietors against loss from any increased price in provisions was to be eliminated. The proprietors were willing to accept these terms on the condition that the by-then familiar clause be inserted into the contract "providing that the insane at the cost and charge of government be not placed elsewhere, while the number in the Beauport Lunatic Asylum is less than 400 now provided for." Although at first resistant to this new "ceiling," the government eventually agreed to the proprietors' request. The new ten-year contract was to take effect on 1 January 1856.[47]

As with previous contracts, the insertion of the ceiling clause, this time giving the Beauport Asylum exclusive rights to government patients up to 400 in number, was crucial to the monopoly status of its proprietors. The legislative allocation for provision for the insane was always completely absorbed by the Beauport Asylum. In other words, the state grant matched the maximum number of patients in the "ceiling clauses" of each contract at Beauport, thus giving the asylum owners complete control over all of the province's government patients. The state frequently increased this legislative allocation in an effort to pressure the Beauport Asylum proprietors to accept a greater number of patients. For example, at the beginning of the 1856–66 contract the state grant for the support of the insane was £10,000. But by 1857 the provincial secretary was already advising that this amount was "insufficient to meet the cost for all applications for admission [to Beauport] from Lower Canada," especially for those from the local jails. The provincial secretary recommended that the state allocation be raised to £12,000 and that the governor general be asked to authorize the necessary admissions from the jails "in anticipation of an increased vote for 1857 as proposed." The increased allowance was quickly approved by the government, and through correspondence with the Beauport proprietors, it was ascertained that an additional thirty-two patients could be received at the asylum by the middle of April 1857. This raised the patient population at Beauport to 400. By 1858, the allocation was increased again to £14,000 and a year later it was set at £15,000, with the Beauport proprietors being asked to take additional patients, increasing the total patient population to 416.[48] Although the ceiling for patients at Beauport had been exceeded, the state still preferred to send "excess" patients to Beauport rather than elsewhere.

By 1861 the number of patients had reached 428, or twenty-eight patients over the official "ceiling clause" in the contract. The overcrowded conditions at the Beauport Asylum were indicative of the increasing demand for asylum accommodation. The government finally responded by establishing the state-controlled St Jean Lunatic Asylum near Montreal in the summer of 1861. By August 1861, the St Jean Asylum was ready to accommodate seventy-two patients. Still, only eight months later, the provincial secretary wrote to Dr Frémont inquiring "how many patients, both male and female" they could "safely admit" at the Beauport Lunatic Asylum.[49] By the time the proprietors' contract was due for renewal in 1864, the asylum population had extended beyond the official "ceiling" of 400 by an additional 150 patients.

Between 1861 and the end of the fourth government contract with the Beauport Lunatic Asylum in 1865, two developments altered the character of subsequent negotiations between the state and the Beauport proprietors. First, reports by the commissioners of the Beauport Lunatic Asylum and by the Board of Inspectors of Asylums, Prisons and Public Charities of the United Canadas (established in 1859) on the negative consequences of patient over-crowding at the Beauport Asylum increased in intensity and in frequency. These reports fuelled the perception among some government officials that there was a need for a greater state presence in the affairs of the Beauport Asylum. The state became particularly interested in involving the Board of Inspectors in negotiations for the renewal of the 1855–65 contract.

The second development was that between 1861 and 1863 Morrin and Frémont both died, leaving James Douglas as the sole proprietor of the Beauport Asylum. In May 1863 with the sanction of the legislature, Douglas entered into partnership with Dr Jean-Etienne Landry, surgeon to the Quebec Marine and Emigrant Hospital, with each physician taking a one-half interest in the asylum. With two of the original proprietors now deceased, negotiations with the state took on a somewhat different character. Although Douglas fought the government over issues of control and power with the same intensity as he and his former co-proprietors had previously done, it was clear that his new partner was more willing to accept an increased state presence at the asylum. This attitude set the relationship between the Beauport Lunatic Asylum and the government on an altered course.

On 13 July 1864, Douglas and Landry petitioned for a renewal of their contract. In a departure from past strategy, the government sent a draft set of terms upon which it would be willing to enter into a new contract with the Beauport Asylum proprietors to the Board of Inspectors of Asylums, Prisons and Public Charities for their review. The government's proposed terms would give the Board of Inspectors increased control over the affairs of the asylum on two fronts. First, the proprietors were to provide suitable accommodation to asylum patients "in such a manner as [would] meet the approval" of the Board of Inspectors. Second, a government-appointed "resident physician" was to be hired at the proprietors' expense to report to the board on the condition of the patients and the asylum.

The Board of Inspectors gave general approval to the terms, but endeavoured to make the proprietors even more accountable to the board. "Any resolutions passed by the Board of Inspectors [in regard to accommodation for asylum patients are] to be acted upon by the proprietors so soon as intimated to them by the Secretary of the Board, notwithstanding any reference or appeal which [the proprietors] may wish to make to the government against it, and will remain good, until the decision of the government in case of such appeal is made known."[50] Moreover, the board requested that the plans of a new building in progress at Beauport be "submitted without delay to His Excellency, the Governor General, for his sanction and [that] such alterations shall be made in any building now in use for the patients, as may be recommended by the said Inspectors, to secure efficient ventilation in the different chambers."[51] This imperative, along with the appointment of a government resident physician, represented a substantial increase in state involvement in the daily affairs of the Beauport Asylum.

During this negotiation between the Board of Inspectors and the government, reports by the Board of Inspectors and Asylum Commissioners on the overcrowded conditions at Beauport continued. Both inspectors and commissioners advised that there were too many patients in the asylum (the number had reached 547 by 1864) and that the accommodation in some of the asylum buildings was in immediate need of improvement.[52] These concerns about overcrowding were crucial to the debate between the proprietors and the state over the maximum number of patients to be set for the new contract. Whereas Douglas and Landry claimed that they had continued new construction at the asylum under the impression that the new "ceiling clause" for patients would be set at 750, both the commissioners of the Beauport Asylum and the Board of Inspectors argued that the overcrowded state of the asylum, as it existed, would only permit the maximum number of patients to be set at 600 upon completion of the construction.

Douglas and Landry were well aware of the significance of the interrelated issues of overcrowding and increased state control on the eve of a contract renewal. In response, they vigorously sought to defend their monopoly. On the subject of overcrowding, Douglas and Landry defended their record on two fronts. First, the Beauport proprietors insisted that they provided adequate "cubic space" for the vast majority of asylum patients at Beauport. Although they concurred that Richardson House, a building for refractory patients, needed to be abandoned and better provision provided for its inhabitants, the proprietors insisted that such an endeavour "would entail upon [them] an amount of expense which the present state of [their] contract would not warrant." Douglas and Landry argued that in reconstructing the centre part of the main building and adding two additional wings to the asylum over the course of the previous year they had spent all funds available for the improvement of accommodation for the insane that the financial terms of their present contract would bear.[53] Second, the proprietors argued that since the beginning of the Beauport Asylum's existence the government had continually "exceeded the estimated wants" of the contract, forcing the proprietors to invest more money in the expansion of the asylum complex. In their opinion, overcrowding was thus the result of state policy and not the fault of the proprietors.[54]

Douglas and Landry also forcefully contested the demand that all asylum architectural plans, including those for the new building for the incurably insane already under construction, were to be sent to the Board of Inspectors for review and possible modification. In the opinion of the proprietors, the Board of Inspectors had been given ample opportunity to examine the plans for the new building before construction had started. They noted that one of the inspectors, Dr Taché, had in fact made some recommendations, and those which "met the approval" of the proprietors had been adopted. The new building, they asserted, was now in such an advanced state of construction that further modification to its structure was impracticable. "We are of opinion that our knowledge and experience enable us to judge more correctly of the wants and requirements of an asylum than any non professional persons [read inspectors!] ... We would remark in conclusion that it would be much easier to alter a plan, than to alter a building should such alteration be deemed necessary." The proprietors, it seemed, would tolerate only limited interference in the construction and design of their asylum.[55]

Beauport's proprietors were especially concerned about the government's intention to appoint its own resident physician to attend to the daily needs of the patients and report on conditions in the asylum. They had previously handpicked their resident physician, a key figure in managing the daily affairs of the Beauport Asylum. Douglas and Landry refused to consider any state-substituted resident physician, especially one whose salary was to be paid for out of their funds.

The government's response to this unqualified resistance on the part of the Beauport proprietors was to change the status of its medical appointment from resident to visiting physician. Although Landry was willing to sign a contract which included this less obtrusive form of state medical appointment, Douglas remained intransigent on the issue. He vented his concern about the proposed physician's role:

The duties and powers of the visiting physician [are still] not defined. He may possess experience and common sense – and he may not be empowered to interfere in the conduct and management of the asylum – in these cases, his appointment would meet the approval of the proprietors, otherwise his appointment would disturb the harmony and the good management which has characterized the Institution during the last twenty years. This management cannot safely be interfered with. If therefore the proposed visiting physician is to be clothed with administrative powers the institution would become a scene of discord and its best interests would suffer.[56]

Douglas protested the appointment of a state medical official to the Beauport Asylum for the very reasons that the state sought such an appointment: increased state inspection and control over the affairs of the institution. In Douglas's view, the consequence would be divided authority in the asylum and compromised care and management of the insane.[57]

By the end of March, negotiations had come to a head. An order-in-council dated 29 March consolidated the government's final position on the conditions of a renewed contract with Douglas and Landry. It recommended that the contract be extended for a term of five years (as opposed to the ten desired by the proprietors). It restricted the number of patients under government contract to a minimum of 550 and a maximum of 650. The duties of the visiting physician remained undefined, but the asylum was to be "accessible to him at all times and in all its ports, as well as to the Commissioners of the Asylum and the Prison Inspectors." The visiting physician was also to "report to the Governor General on the state of the asylum, and on the approval of such report, the proprietors [were] to comply with its requirements." The order-in-council gave the Board of Inspectors the power to cause any "alterations" to be made in "any building now or hereafter in use for the patients ... to secure efficient ventilation in the establishment." A special clause protecting the proprietors in case of war or change of tariff was considered unnecessary, and thus not recommended. Despite Landry's position that the level of state interference enshrined in the order-in-council "leaves us defenceless in the hands of the visiting physician and the Prison Inspectors whom we are obliged to obey *without appeal!*" he grudgingly endorsed its terms, and urged Douglas to do the same. After some further debate, the contract was extended to cover a period of eight years instead of the five years stated in the order-in-council. But the clauses of the contract relating to increased accountability to the state remained much the same. Finally, under much pressure from his partner, Douglas consented to sign.[58]

Douglas remained highly sceptical of the long-term implications of the state's efforts to increase its involvement in the management of the Beauport Asylum. In his opinion, either he and his partner should have unmitigated control over the care of the insane or the "management of so large and so important a public institution ought ... to be in the hands of Government outright." Douglas's main concern thus appeared to be the prospect of divided authority at the Beauport Asylum. After twenty years, the only remaining original proprietor of the Beauport asylum was also tiring of his responsibility in the management and care of the insane. Douglas made it known: "Individually I am anxious to be relieved from so onerous a responsibility, and from so hazardous a risk, and I would refuse no offer which would repay me the cost of the adventure."[59] These sentiments eventually led Douglas to sell his share in the farming-out of lunatics at the Beauport Asylum at the end of December 1865.[60]

Yet, in the final analysis, the state had managed only to a limited extent to wrestle control of the Beauport Asylum out of the hands of its proprietors. Although technically bound by the renewed contract to a more subservient relationship with the Board of Inspectors, the proprietors would clearly tolerate only a low level of interference in the maintenance and physical expansion of their institution. Moreover, through tough contract negotiations, Douglas and Landry had managed to reduce the status of the new state-appointed medical authority at Beauport from that of resident to that of visiting physician. The lively exchanges between the proprietors and the first two visiting physicians, Dr F.E. Roy and Dr A. Jackson, illustrate the relatively minimal impact of state inspection of the insane at Beauport.

In his first reports as a government-appointed visiting physician, Dr Roy focused on the excessive overcrowding at Beauport. His other main concern was the lack of an infirmary for patients who became physically ill during their stay at the asylum.[61] In the late fall of 1865, Roy's inspections led to a much more serious altercation between the proprietors and the state. The conflict centred on whether or not the deaths of two patients in the newly constructed male wing of the asylum were attributable to the excessively cold temperatures in that building. In Roy's recorded observations during the month of October 1865, he repeatedly drew attention to the low temperatures and high humidity in the wards of the new wing. He noted that the heating apparatus was not yet operational in the new wing and that there was insufficient use of stoves to compensate for the lack of heating. In particular, Roy was concerned about patients who refused to keep covered in bed, or those who could not get out of bed and were thus constantly confined to the cold, damp atmosphere. He warned that such patients should be removed to a better-heated area in the asylum. On 27 October he reported that one of the patients whom he had observed to be very ill had died "without being moved to a different cell." and that another was "almost numb with cold." He continued: "I would not like to take on myself the responsibility for allowing this unfortunate person to die in the cold living quarters that he occupies at present."[62]

When this second patient died, Roy's reports were sent to the Board of Inspectors of Prisons, Asylums, and Public Charities for further investigation. After communicating with the proprietors, with the superintendent, and with the resident physician of the asylum, Inspector Taché concluded that the deaths of the two patients were not actually due to the excessive cold in the male wing of the institution, nor to a lack of medical attention on the part of the medical officials. Nevertheless, on the basis of Roy's observations, the government concluded that more attention should have been paid to the temporary heating measures while the permanent apparatus was being installed in the new male wing. The asylum proprietors were strongly advised not to repeat such mistakes in the future.

In his response to the government's reprimand, Landry flatly rejected the visiting physician's criticisms that the new asylum wing was either too cold or too humid. He asserted that stoves had in fact been in operation in the wing during the month of October and that they had provided sufficient heat for the patients. The government maintained its position that its recommendations concerning the proper heating of the asylum were soundly based on the reports of the visiting physician and of the Board of Inspectors. There is no indication that Landry at any stage acknowledged the observations or recommendations of the inspectors.[63]

Perhaps the most symbolic expression of the limited impact of state inspection on the power of the proprietors at Beauport was the quick defection of Dr Roy from his position as state-visiting physician to the status of co-proprietor of the asylum. This defection took place in the context of a larger public scandal surrounding the retirement of James Douglas from his involvement with the Beauport Asylum. Aware of Douglas's dissatisfaction with the terms of the renewed contract of 1865, a member of parliament, M. Cauchon, approached the alienist at an asylum ball with an offer to buy out his interest at Beauport. However, nothing was settled, and Douglas left for Europe the next day. In Douglas's absence, Cauchon approached Douglas's son with an offer of purchase. James Douglas Jr sold part of his father's asylum holdings to Cauchon and the rest to Landry. To avoid any perception of conflict of interest, Cauchon had Roy sign for possession of his part of the deal. Soon afterwards, however, Roy claimed actual ownership of Cauchon's purchase, and in the ensuing scandal, Cauchon was forced to resign his seat "for illegally holding a contract under government."[64] With the knowledge he had gained as visiting physician to the Beauport Asylum, Roy probably came to see the institution as a lucrative professional and business opportunity. As co-proprietor of the Beauport Asylum, Roy became in his turn as vociferous in his denunciation of the next state-appointed visiting physician, Dr Andrew Jackson, as Landry had been of him.[65]

Roy's successful manoeuvre into position as co-proprietor in the farming-out system at Beauport was indicative of the ambitions of many in Quebec during the nineteenth century. There were in fact several proposals between 1840 and 1889 to establish asylums in the lower province on terms similar to those struck between the state and the Beauport proprietors. These proposals indicated two perceptions: that the trade in lunacy as manifested at the Beauport Asylum was a profitable business enterprise; and that many were concerned that the monopoly at Beauport was not serving the needs of the community, or of the insane, in Quebec. These proposals came in the form of public petitions to establish asylums in various communities,[66] and private petitions by individuals wanting to enter into contract with the government for the management and care of the insane.[67]

State officials simply ignored public petitions for asylums. As for petitions issued by private individuals interested in the kind of farming-out system established at the Beauport Lunatic Asylum, the provincial secretary either rejected the proposals outright, or responded in the following way: "The Government would probably avail itself of your proposal for the relief of [the insane] ... were it not that a contract was passed ... with the proprietors of the Asylum near Quebec under the explicit understanding that patients should continue to be sent to their establishment in such number as could cover the amount noted by the legislature for several years past."[68] In other words, the state argued that the "ceiling clause" inserted into each of the contracts with the Beauport proprietors prohibited similar arrangements with any other party. From the point of view of the state, this clause guaranteed that the Beauport Asylum would continue its monopoly over care of government patients.

The government's refusal to entertain any of the great variety of proposals from different quarters suggests that it was in no hurry to alter this monopoly. Although the monopoly was in part the result of shrewd negotiating on the part of Beauport's owners, it is clear that it also suited the needs of the state. The government chose not to push for terms in new contracts that would have enabled it to seek other offers to accommodate the insane. Nor did it choose to move patients in excess of the "ceiling clause" to other institutions as it was legally entitled to do. In its repeated refusal to do either, the government demonstrated its tacit support for Beauport's monopoly position.

Though disinclined to accept any of the many offers of other would-be proprietors, the state was eventually led by pressure from reports on the insufficiency of accommodation for the insane to reconsider the establishment of a provincial or state-controlled asylum in Quebec. Various proposals were tabled to establish a state asylum for the insane on a scale similar to that at Beauport,[69] but the government opted instead for a renovated infantry barracks at St Jean. This site was inspected by Inspector Taché and Joseph Workman, superintendent of the Toronto Provincial Asylum, who deemed it suitable for conversion to an asylum.[70] Renovations of the barracks were supervised by the asylum's appointed superintendent, Dr Henry Howard, and it was ready to accommodate seventy-two patients in August 1861.

Ironically, the St Jean Asylum, over which the state had the full authority and control that it had fought to establish at Beauport, was deemed an inferior institution for the insane both by government inspectors and by its own superintendent. Reports of its inadequacies began immediately after it opened. Poor ventilation, insufficient heating, inadequate centralization of resources, fire hazards, high expenses per patient, and overcrowding were especially noted. Comparisons between St Jean and Beauport inevitably highlighted the comparative superiority of the proprietary institution. According to the chairman of the Board of Inspectors, "We have properly speaking no more than a single asylum. The refuge at St Johns with its 50 beds fills a wretched little Barrack to overflow and cannot be considered an asylum for the insane. Beauport is a fine institution and that is all Lower Canada can boast of."[71]

Superintendent Henry Howard lent his own voice to the criticism of the asylum, frequently proposing the establishment of better accommodation elsewhere.[72] Within a year of its establishment, the St Jean Asylum was relocated to the Old Court House in the city. This move necessitated another period of makeshift renovations and the result, according to the inspectors and Superintendent Howard, was no improvement.[73] Frustrated by the inadequacies of the asylum over which he presided, Howard began to suggest better sites for the public lunatic asylum.[74]

The evident failure of St Jean encouraged further proposals from physicians interested in the farming-out system in Quebec. One proposal was especially noteworthy, as it came from James Douglas, proprietor of Beauport and one of Quebec's most influential doctors, and the well-respected state-appointed superintendent of the Rockwood Criminal Lunatic Asylum in Upper Canada John Palmer Litchfield. Douglas and Litchfield put forth an ambitious offer to establish a large proprietary asylum near Montreal on the grounds of the 300-acre Molson Estate, on the banks of the St Lawrence, with the same relationship to the state as that of Beauport.[75] In their proposal, Douglas and Litchfield highlighted the success of the proprietary arrangement at Beauport, comparing it to the "miserable" record at St Jean. Despite the evident attractiveness of their proposal, the government was ultimately not interested in making a deal with them, possibly out of concern that, as co-proprietor of the Beauport Asylum, Douglas already wielded enough power in the Quebec farming-out system. Moreover, it may have appeared expedient to keep Litchfield in his position as superintendent of the Rockwood Asylum.

When the government was finally pressured into action by inspectors' unfavourable reports on conditions at the St Jean Asylum and by relentless pressure to accommodate more patients, it combined economy and the proprietary model once again – but in a different formula from that of Beauport. In 1873, a contract was struck between the province and the Sisters of Providence to reestablish St Jean de Dieu Asylum at Longue Pointe, about seven miles from Montreal. With the opening of this asylum in 1875, the older St Jean Asylum was closed and its patients were absorbed into the new institution. The contract entered into between the religious order and the state had a twenty-year term, far longer than any contract with the Beauport proprietors.

This arrangement was immensely appealing to the state primarily because the nuns were willing to enter into contracted care of the insane for far less reimbursement than their proprietary lay counterparts at Beauport. The asylum was predominantly staffed by nuns who were not paid in the same way as lay keepers of the insane. Between 1883 and 1887, the difference in cost to the government between the Beauport and St Jean de Dieu asylums averaged $32 per patient per year. The state had found another even more economical means to provide asylum management and care of the insane. As with the original Beauport contract, the initial costs of asylum construction and property purchase were to be shouldered by the Sisters of Providence. The success of this new arrangement from the state's perspective was evidenced by the rapid growth of the patient population at St Jean de Dieu. In 1875 this asylum had 408 patients. By 1884 it had a population of 919, more than Beauport's patient body of 911. Two years later, it was providing for over 1,000 patients.

Although the state was satisfied with the financial arrangements forged with the Beauport and (especially) the St Jean de Dieu asylums, it continued to push for greater control over asylum affairs in both institutions. In the eyes of many state officials, the farming-out system established in Quebec had inherent flaws that necessitated the corrective influence of the state. The Board of Inspectors had been aware of potential conflicts of interest since 1859:

The farming out of lunatics to private persons is in their opinion, as a general rule, most objectionable. In asylums supported by the state, the Medical Superintendent in charge of the Institution has no interest which conflicts with the interests of the patients committed to his care. But in proprietary asylums the case is far otherwise. Here it is plainly the interest of the proprietors or contractors to spend as little as possible on the food and maintenance of the patients, and to get as large a return as possible from them in the shape of labor; on the other hand, it is the interest of the patients that they should be fed liberally, even generously and that they should never be expected, much less compelled, to labor harder or longer than they wish. A system can hardly be expected to work satisfactorily where the interests of the parties concerned are so essentially at variance.

Although the inspectors were quick to point out that at Beauport, "no evils have followed from this defect in the proprietary system," they attributed this degree of success to the "high character of the gentlemen who up to the present time have had the management and control of the Institution." This state of affairs, they implied, could change at any time.[76]

In theory, the religious nature of the proprietary arrangement at the St Jean de Dieu Asylum militated against profiteering at the expense of patients. Nevertheless, the state was determined to regulate the affairs of both institutions more thoroughly. The Inspectors of

Asylums in Quebec argued: "The system followed in this province with respect to the support of the insane, while having the advantage of being less expensive, is not nearer perfection than the system usually followed in other countries, but it is not so very defective as to prevent its being made good use of and the patients from being treated as well and with as good chances of success as elsewhere."[77] In the inspectors' opinion, if the farming-out system was accompanied by a strong state influence, the province could reap the benefits of inexpensive care of the insane while at the same time guaranteeing high standards in the management and organization of the province's asylums.

Unable to negotiate by contract for increased state involvement in either asylum, the state eventually endeavoured to exercise its regulatory powers through legislative means. Thus in 1885 An Act Relating to Insane Asylums in the Province of Quebec was passed, for the better management of lunatic asylums in Quebec. The central feature of the act of 1885 was the creation of state Medical Boards to regulate the asylums at Beauport and Longue Pointe.[78] The Medical Boards were each composed of three physician inspectors: a visiting physician, a house physician, and an assistant house physician. The visiting and house physicians were state-appointed, and their salaries were paid by the government. According to this law, the asylum proprietors could choose their own assistant house physician but would in that case be responsible for his salary. Alternatively they could leave the assistant house physician's appointment to the state, in which case his salary, like those of the other two physicians on the medical board, would be paid by the government. However, even if the proprietors chose their own assistant house physician, the appointment still had to meet the approval of the Lieutenant Governor-in-Council.

In effect, the Medical Board constituted the state's attempt to exercise full supervision and control over the medical affairs and several other aspects of both institutions. The asylums were to be accessible to the Medical Board at all times; its physicians were to make full reports to the government on the state of the institutions; and the recommendations made by the Medical Board in regard to asylum management and care were to be legally binding on the asylums' proprietors. Under the law, the house physician or assistant house physician was empowered to dismiss keepers and nurses, subject to the approval of the inspector of asylums.[79]

The proprietors of both asylums vigorously opposed the passage of the 1885 law and after it had passed, did all they could to thwart the increased state influence that the new law prescribed. Even as the legislation was being tabled by government, the proprietors of the Beauport and St Jean de Dieu asylums argued that the new law constituted a violation of the contracts they held with the state. Within the terms of their respective contracts, both institutions did everything in their power to deny the authority vested in the Medical Boards by the state. For example, the doctors of the Medical Boards were treated by the proprietors of both institutions strictly as visiting physicians, whose presence the proprietors tolerated only at appointed times and only in the company of asylum employees designated by the proprietors. The physicians of the Medical Boards were also frequently denied access to information they needed for their reports to the government. Finally, the proprietors in both institutions prohibited asylum employees from answering the questions of the Medical Boards or from giving the board physicians information pertinent to their government reports.[80]

The resistance to the Act of 1885 by both institutions reflected fundamental differences between the proprietors and the state in regard to the state's role in the management and care of the insane. Since its founding in 1845, the Beauport Asylum proprietors had fought vigorously to exclude the presence of the state from the affairs of the institution. This was in part due simply to the proprietary nature of the asylum. As mid-nineteenth-century businessmen, Beauport's owners ran the asylum with the full intention of profiting from the endeavour. Profits were most effectively achieved without undue interference from the state. This attitude reflected prevailing liberal ideas on the role of the state in enterprise.

Beauport's proprietors were also concerned about the consequences of divided authority in their institution. All nineteenth-century lunatic asylums, whether private or state-run, tended to be very hierarchical in their organization. Douglas and his associates had ample opportunity to witness the negative consequences of authority clashes in the publicly run asylums in the neighbouring province of Ontario, and elsewhere. It is likely that such evidence further convinced Beauport's proprietors that absolute control in the farming-out system generated the best results. Finally, it is apparent that for most of the period from 1845 to 1888 the

Beauport Asylum's owners were convinced that they ran a world-class institution for the insane. Their success, they argued, had been achieved from the outset with a minimal amount of state interference in the management and organization of their undertaking. They saw no need to introduce such interference, especially from an inspectorate whose accumulated expertise and experience they considered no match for their own.

The religious proprietors' response to the Act of 1885 demonstrated that they were no less resistant to the idea of state interference in the conduct of their institution. But in the case of the St Jean de Dieu Asylum, hostility to the Act of 1885 stemmed in large measure from traditional Catholic perceptions in Quebec of the role of the state in society. According to the Bishop of Three Rivers, the Act of 1885 was "founded on the false principle of the omnipotence of the State," an error which had led to the "over-throw of all the religious institutions of France, our old mother-country." The Bishop argued that the state "had no right to assume [the] management and control, nor to infringe upon the rights of property and canonical immunity" of any of the religious institutions of Quebec, be they Hôtels-Dieu, seminaries, convents, or asylums for the insane. Such rights were assumed by the Sisters of Providence when they entered into contract with the state for the care of the insane at Longue Pointe. Several other Quebec bishops supported this position.[81] This line of argument, of course, was about much more than specific concerns over the running of a particular institution. It formed part of the larger struggle between the Catholic Church and the state in nineteenth-century Quebec. It also reflected contrasting views on the role of benevolent institutions in the care and treatment of the insane and differences of opinion between the state and the Catholic Church on the definition of insanity.

The impasse created by the resistance of the proprietors at the Beauport and St Jean De Dieu asylums to the Act of 1885 eventually led to the establishment of a Royal Commission on Lunatic Asylums of the Province of Quebec in 1887.[82] The primary mandate of the Royal Commission was to determine whether the Act of 1885 infringed on the legal rights of asylum proprietors as delineated in their respective contracts with the government. The commissioners concluded that in some respects, especially in regard to the powers invested in the Medical Boards, the state had in fact overstepped the limits of its legal rights of asylum inspection and control.[83]

Another important aspect of the Royal Commission's mandate was to investigate the extent to which the asylums in Quebec were kept in a "satisfactory condition," given the money spent by the government for their maintenance. The commissioners in general praised the work of the Sisters of Providence in the superior maintenance of their institution at the low cost of $100 per patient per year. They attributed their success to the fact "that the asylum is under the constant superintendence of a staff composed almost entirely of nuns ... from the humble lay sister to the Lady Superior in whom is vested supreme authority." Their main criticism of the Sisters' asylum was that its medical staff was neither large enough nor powerful enough to make the changes within the institution "now considered indispensable by science, both as regards classification and treatment." The commissioners also strongly urged that the medical staff be completely accountable to the state.[84]

The commissioners' review of the Beauport Asylum was comparatively unflattering. They noted that, given the rate of $132 per patient per year charged by the proprietors, the quality of the medical service at Beauport was very poor, the superintendence by the keepers of the institution was neglected to the point that the "comfort, health and safety of the patients" was constantly wanting, and the food and clothing of the patients left much to be desired.[85] In their judgment, the Beauport proprietors had not fulfilled the conditions of their contract, and accordingly, it ought to be cancelled. They concluded that the best solution to the problems at Beauport would be for the government to hand over the "internal administration" of the asylum to a religious community whose powers would be confined "exclusively to the domestic and administrative management" of the institution. "For everything relating to the treatment of the patients" the commissioners recommended that "the nuns should have to rely solely upon a competent medical staff responsible to the Government."[86]

As in previous clashes between the state and the proprietors of Quebec's lunatic asylums, the message of the Royal Commission was clear: the government demanded increased influence and control over the affairs of Beauport and St Jean de Dieu. But by 1888 there had been a noticeable change in the government's strategy for achieving its aims. Although still expressing concern over the farming-out system, the state had obviously come to see a particular form of this system – contracts with religious orders in Quebec – as by far the cheapest means to furnish institutional provision for the insane. However, the role of the religious organizations was to be restricted to the "caring" aspects of asylum provision, leaving the medical and administrative responsibilities to a board of physicians that held "absolute powers" and that was to be appointed by and accountable to the state.[87]

In certain respects, the 1887 Royal Commission and its consequences represented a victory for the state in the struggle to control institutional management of insanity in Quebec. In 1890, with the opening of the Verdun Protestant Hospital for the Insane, the provincial government gained complete control over the medical treatment of the asylum. In 1893, when the Beauport Asylum contract expired, the institution was sold to the Sisters of Charity of Quebec, who, by law, forfeited medical control of the asylum to the government-appointed Medical Board. The Sisters contracted with the government to care for patients at $100 per year per head. Finally, although it was to be somewhat less successful in its renewal of the contract with the St Jean de Dieu Asylum in 1897, the province managed to establish an arrangement whereby physicians chosen by the Sisters of Providence would work alongside state-appointed medical officials.[88]

An interesting comparison can be drawn between nineteenth-century developments in the institutional care and management of the insane in Quebec and in France. Historian Jan Goldstein notes that, starting in the early seventeenth century, religious congregations in France had actively embarked upon a mission in the care of the insane. The French Revolution put an abrupt end to this enterprise, but it flourished again during the Restoration Period. Thus, "a massive early nineteenth-century expansion of religious facilities for the insane coincided with the emergence of a scientific *médicine mentale* – a pattern," Goldstein asserts, that "must cast doubt on any theory postulating a uniformly rising curve of professionalization, modernization, or secularization."[89] Goldstein argues that in France the tradition of "religious consolation" used in the institutional care of the insane by the religious orders was so similar in theory and in practice to the moral treatment advocated by asylum alienists that the psychiatric profession had great difficulty in asserting its expertise in the diagnosis, treatment, and management of insanity.[90] The French state was therefore content to deal with religious orders in the institutional provision for the insane. It was not until the end of the nineteenth century that French alienists became sufficiently professionalized to decisively wrest control of the treatment and care of the insane from the religious orders. A contributing factor in the increasing domination of the psychiatric profession was a professional/political alliance with the French state during the last decades of the nineteenth century.[91]

The historical development of relations between the state and the Catholic Church in the management of insanity in Quebec was in many respects the opposite of that in France. To the extent that state-financed institutional provision for the insane existed in early nineteenth-century Quebec, it was provided by religious orders in the *système des loges,* a tradition that had started early in the eighteenth century in New France. Over the course of the nineteenth century, mounting criticism of the *loges* was coupled with the growing sense that the lunatic asylum was the proper environment for the treatment and management of insanity. In its efforts to rationalize the call for asylum treatment of insanity with the financial constraints of its colonial setting, the state opted for a proprietary and secular arrangement which quickly turned into a monopoly in asylum care and treatment of the insane in Quebec – a monopoly that went virtually uncontested until the mid-1870s. But, just as religious orders in France were losing their control over the institutional "consolation" of the insane, religious orders in Quebec began to dominate the general management of lunatic asylums – a testimony both to the relative influence of the Church in the province and to the state's desire to further reduce expenditure in this branch of its activities. However, although religious orders maintained tremendous influence on the everyday management and care of the insane, in the late nineteenth century the Quebec government finally managed to impose state regulation on medical treatment and administration within asylums. This particular combination of religious-based "care" and state-controlled secular "medicine" was the hallmark of a relationship between insanity and the state that was unique to Quebec. The situation that emerged in Ontario was very different.

2 Insanity, Community and Commissioner: The State and the Government System in Ontario

In his study of the history of the hospital in the United States, Charles Rosenberg points out the "inconsistent visions" of hospital physicians and trustees in the nineteenth century. He notes that although trustee and physician agreed "on matters of class definition and the social styles appropriate to these definitions" as they pertained to the hospital, disputes between them frequently resulted from the physician's more medical conception of hospital practice.[1]

In the lunatic asylums of nineteenth-century Ontario, inconsistent visions also existed among medical superintendent, asylum commissioner, and, later, asylum inspector. But the conflicts that arose between medical and lay officials of the nineteenth-century Ontario asylum differed from those uncovered by Rosenberg for the hospital setting in the United States. Most asylum superintendents had a vision of the state asylum that corresponded closely to concepts of the ideal institution for the treatment and regulation of insanity described in prevailing medical literature and promoted by asylum advocates. They were influenced by prominent writers on this subject such as American alienist Thomas Kirkbride, whose "Kirkbride model" of asylum architecture and organization was highly influential in Canada. They envisioned the lunatic asylum as an institution in which the authority of the physician superintendent reigned supreme and the architecture and internal management were carefully shaped for the practice of medical and moral therapy. During the period of the temporary lunatic asylum in Toronto from 1840 to 1850, this vision contrasted sharply with that of the asylum commissioners, who did not share the superintendents' medical or moral outlook. Shortly after the opening of the permanent lunatic asylum in 1850, the balance between views about asylum care shifted, but differences in perspective between superintendent and inspector persisted, culminating in serious conflicts that had a major impact on the development of the state institution.

Community perceptions about what services an asylum should offer also differed markedly from the therapeutic ideals of medical superintendents. Dissension arose among local, asylum, and government officials as to whose interests the state institution would ultimately serve and the kind of institution that should eventually emerge. Concerns relating to the financing of the state institution also influenced the overall character of the asylum. Difficulty in raising funds to construct and maintain the province's public asylums consistently compromised the respective visions of government inspectors, medical superintendents, and community members.

State management and treatment of the mentally ill in Ontario did not really begin until the establishment of a provisional asylum in 1840. Prior to that time the insane in Upper Canada had been provided for mainly within their local community or in county jails. In 1830 an act was passed legalizing the practice of payment for the maintenance of the insane in Toronto's Home District Jail, and in 1833 it was amended to include all districts in Upper Canada.[2] The incarceration of the insane with jail inmates caused overcrowding in local jails and drew heavy criticism in grand jury reports and from jail wardens. Their concerns about mixing various problem groups under one roof echoed those voiced in Quebec.[3] Between the 1833 legislation and the establishment of the temporary lunatic asylum in Toronto in 1840, several legislative initiatives were tabled for the institutional care of the insane but, for both political and practical reasons, all of them failed.[4]

In 1839, legislation was finally passed granting £3,000 towards the establishment of a permanent lunatic asylum. The act called for the appointment of government commissioners to supervise the construction of the asylum. Upon completion of the asylum, the government was to appoint a twelve-member board of directors with powers to establish rules and regulations for the effective management of the institution. The board would also be empowered to appoint all medical and lay employees to the asylum. Each district was to pay an annual asylum tax of "one eighth of a penny to the pound," to be used towards "the erection of the ... Asylum, and in the purchasing of land sufficient for a site, and maintaining and supporting the same."[5]

As in Quebec, the pressure to make provisional arrangements for the insane while awaiting the construction of a permanent asylum led to the renovation of the old Home District Jail for use as a temporary lunatic asylum in 1840.[6] However, unlike its Lower Canada counterpart, the Toronto Temporary Lunatic Asylum remained in operation for a full decade until the official opening of a permanent asylum in 1850.

This asylum represented the efforts of the Upper Canada government to develop a state institution based on the principles of medical science, state inspection, and regulation. To this end, Dr William Rees, a long-time proponent of state-controlled institutional care for the insane in Upper Canada, was appointed superintendent of the temporary asylum.[7] The Honourable R.S. Jamieson, W.B. Jarvis, Dr W.C. Gwynne, and John Ewart were appointed commissioners for the management of the asylum, and by 1843 the number of commissioners had increased to twelve.[8] In 1842 the government called upon the commissioners to draft a code of rules and regulations for the "internal management" of the asylum that would outline the duties and responsibilities of each institution officer. In describing their own roles, the commissioners defined themselves as gratuitously appointed government inspectors and general managers of the asylum. Their duties included attending weekly meetings, looking into "the state of the institution and condition of the patients, hearing all complaints, [making] tenders for contracts, examining accounts, and generally taking cognizance of all matters concerned with the institution." One of the commissioners was to visit the asylum on a daily basis to ensure that patients were being treated properly and to consult with the superintendent on asylum matters. The commissioners were to submit an anual report of their observations on the financial footing and general state of the institution. According to the rules and regulations, the medical superintendent had charge of the "internal management of the institution as well as the well-being of the patients." The superintendent was to visit the asylum at least three times a day to give directions for medical treatment of the patients and to ensure that the "moral government" of the institution was properly enforced. It was his duty to keep daily records of patient diet, patient medical history, and prescribed medical treatments. As well as attending the commissioners' weekly meetings he was to submit to them an annual report on the state of the institution.

The rules and regulations also gave the asylum steward considerable power and responsibility. Although subject to the control of the medical superintendent, he was responsible for ensuring that all the superintendent's directives in regard to the medical and moral treatment of patients were successfully carried out. To execute this responsibility effectively, the steward was to remain at the asylum unless given the superintendent's permission to leave. The steward was responsible for the cleanliness of the male patients, the quality of the food, the patients' clothing, the asylum furniture, and the maintenance of the building exterior. He had the authority to appoint and dismiss "ordinary servants" of the institution and, under the direction of the commissioners and medical superintendent, to hire and be responsible for the asylum's male keepers (or attendants). The steward was not empowered, however, to dismiss attendants without the permission of the commissioners. Upon request, he was to attend the meetings of the commissioners, and keep minutes of the proceedings; and he could be called upon to give assistance in the female ward when needed.

The matron of the asylum followed the steward in the chain of responsibility and authority. She was responsible for the general "house keeping" of the institution, including patient cleanliness, asylum sanitation and good order, and the proper preparation and delivery of meals. She was also responsible for the safekeeping of all articles belonging to the institution and the personal possessions of the female patients. In conjunction with the commissioners and medical superintendent, she could hire attendants and, like the steward, needed the commissioners' approval to dismiss them. Below these high-ranking officers were the head nurse, porter, attendants or keepers of the insane, and ordinary servants.[9]

The asylum rules and regulations were designed to establish a definite institutional hierarchy. This hierarchy, grounded in existing class and gender power relations, was intended to create an efficient and rational environment in which to restore reason to the insane. Through it, the state could monitor the internal affairs of the asylum, assess its performance, and direct policy accordingly. The asylum was "panoptic", in Foucault's sense of the term, insofar as it was designed to function through this chain of authority to inform the state of the performance of its institution. The commissioners' rules and regulations corresponded to the broader goals of the nineteenth-century state lunatic asylum; that is, to control madness through the application of asylum medicine and impart to the insane the institutionalized values of the asylum's bourgeois advocates.

Although the rules and regulations governing the Toronto Temporary Lunatic Asylum expressed the nineteenth-century concept of an ideal asylum, the infrastructure that was expected to accompany those rules was lacking. In reality, the Toronto Temporary Lunatic Asylum was not an archetypical asylum in the way David Rothman has defined it.[10] It had neither a central administrative building nor highly organized patient wings that would have allowed classification of the insane according to disposition or malady. Nor did it embody the architectural symmetry or internal organization that the commissioners considered vital to the regulation and cure of insanity by asylum superintendents.[11] The exercise of moral therapy, as defined by the philosophy of the nineteenth-century state asylum, was also impossible, given the architectural constraints of the renovated jail. There was no "architecture as therapy" to accompany the social organization envisioned for the new asylum in its rules and regulations.[12]

Financial difficulties compounded the architectural and internal failings of the fledgling state institution. Within a year of its opening, members of the grand jury and asylum officials expressed their concern that the institution was "languishing for want of the necessary support to maintain its existence." Insufficient funding plagued the provisional asylum for most of its ten-year existence, with resulting shortages in monies for supplies, employee salaries, and the government's maintenance of pauper patients in the institution.[13]

A prolonged series of major disputes among the senior officers of the asylum further contributed to its failings as an ideal state institution. Conflicts between the asylum commissioners and successive medical superintendents were especially rancorous. These clashes were of major importance as they arose out of conflicting views among the institution's authorities over the significance of the new state institution. A close analysis of the disputes at the upper echelons of the asylum hierarchy during the period 1843 to 1853 shows that the Toronto Temporary Asylum was really a transitional institution that embodied, at once, both traditional and newer ideas about the purposes of a state institution. Early conflicts between asylum superintendents and commissioners reveal that the commissioners did not consider their role in the moral regulation of insanity to be their primary duty. As the ultimate authorities over a large public institution, the commissioners saw in their privileged positions many opportunities for increased political and financial leverage through the strategic dispensation of patronage. The asylum superintendents, in contrast, appear to have embraced an understanding of their role as regulators of insanity through the mechanisms of the state institution over which they presided – an understanding more closely tied to the newer philosophy of the state institution. These differences in perspective were not resolved until the tenure of Joseph Workman as superintendent of the permanent Toronto Lunatic Asylum after 1853. Workman's career as superintendent marks a definite shift in the nature of the lunatic asylum in Ontario.

Outward signs of conflict between commissioners and superintendent began with the publication of a grand jury report on the state of the asylum in the spring of 1844. Based on a discussion with Superintendent Rees, the jurors reported: "The superintendent physician complains (and it seems correctly) that the other officers of the establishment (the Steward and keepers) are not under his control, and are not therefore compelled to obey him, or to cooperate with him; and there is consequently an antagonism between himself and the officers of the institution which impairs its efficiency and which it is feared may be hurtful to the interests of the unhappy beings who are subjected to its management as well as to the pecuniary interests of the establishment."[14] Rees's complaint about an "absence of controlling power and authority" in the asylum became the central focus of debate between him and the commissioners of the institution. The commissioners demanded of Rees further elaboration of his statements to the grand jury. In response, Rees gave several examples of the insubordination of the steward, who, he was quick to point out, was supposedly subject to the superintendent's authority according to the rules and regulations of the asylum.

One example, a dispute between Rees and Steward Napleton, centred on the patient A. Johnson, a man of "highly respectable character." In response to Johnson's complaints about the noise made by patients around him, Rees ordered that he be kept in the room designated for the weekly meetings of the commissioners, there being no other rooms available in the asylum. Rees further ordered that no strangers were to be admitted into the room during Johnson's convalescence. According to Rees these orders had been delivered to the steward, who in turn had forwarded them to the commissioners. Yet, on several occasions thereafter, the steward defied the superintendent's orders by entertaining his personal acquaintances in the room. Rees argued that the exposure of the patient to "society admitted to the room" aggravated Johnson's insanity. In one instance, Johnson was apparently removed from the room and allowed to wander into the female ward, where the superintendent found him "in a very irritable and excited state."

Another conflict emerged when Rees, with the sanction of the chairman of the Board of Commissioners, hired a new attendant to help with one of the more intractable patients in the asylum. Napleton, not having himself heard from the commissioners about the new hiring, refused to acknowledge the new attendant as an employee of the institution. According to Rees, the best solution to this particular difficulty was to give him, as superintendent, the independent power to hire and dismiss attendants and other low-ranking asylum officers. Rees was further upset by Napleton's habit of taking patients into the city for the day. In one such instance, against Rees's expressed wishes, Napleton took a patient to the residences of two of the asylum commissioners and then to a concert of the St George Society in the city. Rees also charged Napleton with inviting visitors on tours of the asylum and with "misrepresent[ing] and prejudic[ing] the minds of the visitors" about the kind of medical treatment practised by the superintendent.[15]

Although Rees's accusations of insubordinate behaviour on the part of the asylum steward did not constitute a direct critique of the commissioners themselves, they did implicate the commissioners indirectly. Rees in effect asserted that, despite their awareness of the defiance of the steward towards him, the commissioners had done nothing to correct this unfortunate state of affairs. Moreover, he claimed that as the highest public officers in authority at the asylum, the commissioners were ultimately responsible for the smooth running of the institution that was badly in want of "a controlling power."

In their report on Rees's complaints, the commissioners played down the instances of insubordination recounted in the superintendent's letter. They implied that the grand jury report that had precipitated the original dispute was largely based on dubious information provided by Rees, which tended to "excite public distrust of the institution and censure upon the Board." They were particularly reluctant to devolve to the superintendent the power to hire and dismiss keepers and nurses, a power that they claimed to be ready to use in the event that Rees had any *legitimate* objection to the conduct of a particular attendant of the asylum. Finally, the commissioners noted that Rees had "for a long time by complaints and accusations which your committee find to be groundless, disturbed the harmony that ought to exist between himself and both the Steward and the Commissioners."[16] The message was clear: the superintendent alone was responsible for any discord emanating from the temporary asylum.

Within a year relations between Superintendent Rees and the commissioners had taken a definite turn for the worse. In a letter to the provincial secretary, Rees noted the asylum attendants' complete defiance of his orders. In order to re-establish authority in the institution, Rees again requested that the power to hire and dismiss asylum attendants be removed from the hands of the commissioners and be vested in the authority of the superintendent. He also complained that the asylum's provisions were being acquired through contracts that the steward had awarded to several of the commissioners.[17] According to Rees, this collusion between the steward and the commissioners had caused financial loss to the asylum and proved that the network of insubordination within the institution could be traced to the commissioners themselves.

In response, the Board of Commissioners argued that "the great and almost sole difficulty" with which they had to contend in the management of the institution was the fact that the asylum's rules and regulations were "completely ineffectual" under Rees's control.

Far from granting Rees more power within the institution, they recommended that the superintendent's power be diminished through
the appointment of consulting and visiting physicians who "should
have control over the medical superintendent in the treatment of
the patients." They argued that this recommendation was necessary
in light of recent complaints by friends of asylum patients that
Rees's medical treatment was unnecessarily severe.[18] Rees coun-
tered that the major impediment to the successful management of
the temporary asylum thus far had been the "lack" of power
accorded to the superintendent. Quoting the renowned alienists
Philippe Pinel and Etienne Esquirol, Rees argued the case for the
supreme rule of the superintendent in the asylum over which he
presided.[19]

   The impasse between Rees and the commissioners finally came to
a head when the provincial secretary made it clear that there was
"no alternative but either to dispose with [the services of the superintendent or] lose the services of the commissioners of the asylum."
Recognizing the threat to his own career, Rees issued an apology for
his statements in his letter to the provincial secretary. In their
response to Rees's overture, the commissioners completely undermined the authority of the superintendent: they accepted his apology but at the same time recommended that he be demoted to the
status of resident physician. A consulting physician would be chosen by the commissioners to "superintend and control the medical
department of the institution until the permanent asylum be complete and established."[20] Before the decision of the Board of Commissioners could be put into effect, Rees suffered a series of physical injuries that forced his retirement from the asylum.

Rees's successor, Dr Telfer, was also party to a series of disputes
with the commissioners. In the spring of 1848, the commissioners
reported to the government that an investigation of a committee of
the board had found Telfer to be completely unfit to fulfill his
duties as superintendent. They accused him of being occasionally
inebriated while on duty at the asylum, of treating some of his
patients with undue harshness, of using the medicines of the institution for his own use in private practice, and of pilfering food supplies from the asylum. Noting that these practices were "destructive
of respect towards [the office of superintendent] amongst the other
officers and the servants of the institution, and of confidence

amongst [themselves]," the commissioners called for the immediate dismissal of the superintendent.[21] The government quickly acceded to their request.

When informed of the investigation, and of his dismissal from office, Telfer demanded that the government allow him to see the evidence upon which the accusations had been made. He assured the provincial secretary that a full and "impartial" investigation would prove him innocent of all charges. He was particularly outraged by not having been made aware of the investigation or having been allowed to account for the claims against him. He accused the commissioners of contracting with a corrupt steward who made exorbitant profits while supplying the asylum. Telfer forwarded letters in his defence from various officers of the asylum (including Dr Primrose, his interim replacement as superintendent) who attested to his good character while pointing out the corrupt practices of the steward and the matron.[22] But once its decision had been made, the government was not prepared to grant Telfer the judicial inquiry he requested. "The true question which concerns the public is not whether you are culpable, to the whole extent of the charges imputed to you, but whether the government which is responsible for your performance of your duty in a highly important position can continue the confidence necessary to [keep you in office]." A full inquiry, the provincial secretary added, would have the undesirable result of putting the integrity of the Board of Commissioners into question.[23]

In a private letter to the provincial secretary, one of the commissioners, the Reverend John Roaf, anticipating that an inquiry would lead to the dismissal of Telfer, requested that John Scott, his son-in-law, take over as superintendent.[24] Despite this pre-emptive endorsement, however, Scott was not appointed and the position was given to Dr George Park, brother-in-law to the Honourable Dr John Rolph.

Soon after Park's appointment, conflicts between the superintendent and the commissioners arose in much the same way as they had with Telfer and Rees. However, Park was much more vociferous than his predecessors in his battle with the commissioners. His voluminous remonstrances against the commissioners exemplify even more clearly the fundamental differences of opinion between superintendent and commissioners on the role of the lunatic asylum as a state institution.

Within four months of his appointment as superintendent, George Park complained to the government about "an antagonism ... between the commissioners and the medical superintendent, which must necessarily be productive of evil results." Park noted that the antagonism hinged on the commissioners' refusal to grant his requests for the discharge of keepers and other asylum servants who were insubordinate to the superintendent and negligent in their duties. He asserted that when charges against attendants were made, the accused "repaired to their favourite commissioner to make interest against the superintendent, steward, or matron," returning to the asylum with "an air of defiance which [was] anything but satisfactory." According to Park, the asylum's patients were made "a matter of secondary consideration, to that of a paltry patronage to keepers, and servants, vigorously exercised by the commissioners." In a now familiar argument, he reiterated that the best solution to this unfortunate state of affairs was to vest the power of appointment and dismissal of such officers in the medical superintendent.[25]

Park was especially angered by the commissioners' consistent refusal to dismiss asylum attendants. Difficulties had begun during the temporary superintendentship of Dr John Rolph, who occasionally replaced Park during the latter's absence from the institution. Rolph discovered a letter to Commissioner Roaf, in which an attendant named Hungerford reported that Jane Hamilton, a female attendant, who was unwell and not able to continue work at the asylum, was being recommended for dismissal by the matron and the steward. Hungerford wrote that several of the asylum attendants and servants objected to Hamilton's dismissal and that Hamilton herself was asking for the protection of Commissioner Roaf in the matter. Rolph's reaction was that in defying the wishes of a senior officer of the asylum and in acting as "the communicant of jealousies" among the employees of the institution, Hungerford was acting in an insubordinate manner completely inappropriate for an attendant. Rolph also asserted that Hungerford had previously been cautioned for being under the influence of liquor while on duty and for smoking tobacco while in the presence of patients in the asylum attic. Rolph therefore suspended Hungerford from service at the asylum pending a meeting of the Board of Commissioners on the subject.[26]

At the meeting Rolph presented his testimony against Hungerford, asking for his dismissal from service. According to Rolph, the commissioners responded by intimating to him that "the dismissal of Hungerford would place the Board in the awkward situation of throwing discredit on the [attendant] whose evidence" had been relied on to effect the dismissal of Park's predecessor, Superintendent Telfer.[27] The commissioners reprimanded Hungerford for writing the letter and reinstated him as attendant. Certain that Hungerford's return would compromise "the good internal government of the institution," Rolph immediately suspended the attendant again and called for his dismissal at the next meeting of the commissioners. In response to Rolf's persistence, the commissioners finally decided to suspend Hungerford from the asylum on full pay until the return of Superintendent Park.[28]

On Park's return, he was as insistent as Rolph had been that Hungerford was not an appropriate attendant for service at the asylum. He therefore ordered the steward to suspend the attendant yet again. But the steward refused to obey Park's order. Park then gave his own order for the attendant to leave the asylum. Hungerford left, only to return a short time later "with instructions ... from Commissioner O'Bierne to maintain his position in the institution in defiance" of Park's orders. Park then called on a group of attendants to "turn" Hungerford out of the asylum. In response to Park's stubbornness, the commissioners issued a punitive decree to all officers of the asylum: they were "to obey the medical superintendent in all that relate[d] to the patients, but ... in all other matters they would be required to obey the Board only."[29]

The commissioners' decree significantly reduced the power of the medical superintendent. Park's response indicates the extent to which the asylum's difficulties hinged upon a struggle for power between the superintendent and the commissioners: When once appointed, I [considered employees of the asylum] also my servants, not merely yours. You may have the right of confirming appointments: but the moment you place them in the position of keepers and publish them in your regulations as subject to my orders, you can have no power to overrule my proceedings with them in my official duties, without transcending the bounds of your commission, invading the more important sphere assigned to me and wounding the high authority under which we all act." In an extraordinary action, Park suspended the steward and all the asylum attendants who were responsible to him, and turned to the "Magistracy and the Police" for help in managing the institution until the government was in a position to "redeem the institution from its anarchy."[30]

The impasse created by the escalation of conflict between the commissioners and the superintendent led to an investigation by the Executive Council in government. The government concluded that the rules and regulations of the temporary asylum ultimately vested supreme authority for the hiring and firing of asylum officers in the commissioners. Park did not have the authority to repeatedly suspend Hungerford in defiance of the orders of the commissioners. The government was more concerned, however, by the broader state of discord that the dispute over Hungerford had illustrated. On this issue the government was much more sympathetic to the superintendent. It expressed its dismay that an attendant whom the superintendent had frequently deemed unfit for asylum work had been consistently reinstated by the commissioners. The executive committee also warned that "a vigourous exertion of authority on the part of the commissioners over the servants of the establishment" was called for, in order to enforce "deference towards the superintendent and harmony of action amongst themselves." The commissioners and superintendent were urged to cooperate in bringing the asylum into "a proper state of order and discipline" before the impending transfer of the asylum to its permanent location.[31]

The commissioners responded by refuting and dismissing all of the superintendent's complaints against them. They were indignant that "after so long and gratuitous a discharge of onerous and disagreeable duties" the government would continue to keep employed a superintendent who "in his communications with the Governor General, [had] so slandered those in whose hands the management of the asylum [had] been placed." The commissioners made it clear that as long as Park still held "the confidence of the government" they saw no option but to resign. But in this case, the government was prepared neither to dismiss Park nor to accept the resignation of the Board. Noting that the recommendations of the executive council were in fact justified, it insisted that the commissioners endeavour to fulfil their role in restoring order to the asylum.[32]

In the following weeks, the state of conflict between the commissioners and Park intensified with the outbreak of more controversies involving other attendants, rules and procedures, and certain aspects of the superintendent's medical practice.[33] Finally, on 20 December 1848, the commissioners reiterated to the government their inability to communicate with Park and again strongly recommended his dismissal from office. This time the Executive Council saw no option but to dismiss Park, although they made it clear that their decision "involve[d] neither a condemnation nor an acquittal of either party as respect[ed] the matter put in issue between them."[34]

George Park did not consider his dismissal to be an end to the controversy between himself and the commissioners. In an eighty-page defence of his short career as superintendent of the temporary lunatic asylum, he described in strong language what he considered to be the gross negligence of the asylum's commissioners in the performance of their duties. Park emphasized the similarities between his experience and that of Drs Telfer and Rees before him in an effort to make a broader set of arguments to explain the problems at the temporary asylum. In the following passage, the wider social and political context in which Park set his critique of the Board of Commissioners begins to emerge:

Throughout the suffering history of the country, the scourge of the magistracy, (ever holding their "onerous and gratuitous offices" from the crown, with perfect immunity from the punishment of their oppressions) was keenly felt and daily complained of without redress. And the aristocratic Commissioners of the Asylum, empowered with their keepers, to beat, bruise, straight jacket and incarcerate in cells the defenceless Lunatics, ought to be regarded with no corrupt partiality; but the same principles of honor, justice and good faith should have been equally extended to me and the inmates, as to the Board. How did the inmates in the Penitentiary in Kingston suffer from their Commissioners "with their onerous and gratuitous services"? How long they suffered, at their irresponsible hands, flagellations of body and deteriorations of mind, because *gentlemen* and *priests* could not be supposed to do wrong, or be subjected to the *low practice* of being *called to an account*; inasmuch as such democratic conduct towards them would astound our reform government with the dreadful threat of a "resignation." In truth, the Penitentiary ... and the Asylum have fallen, from the same objectionable policy, into the same condition; those in the former have relief because seen and heard by their friends, while those in the latter are doomed to unchanging hands, because uncredited in their appeals and unsupported by the sympathy of those, who have literally converted an *Asylum* into a *prison*, upon whose threshold comparatively few have ever deigned to cast their shadow, or have power or influence to afford redress.[35] [Emphasis added.]

It is obvious that Park aimed to cast the commissioners in as unfavourable a light as possible. Yet, personal hostility aside, his critique brings into sharp relief the differing principles upon which superintendents and commissioners based their respective views of the asylum.

The 1849 Brown Commission into the state of affairs at the Kingston Penitentiary, to which Park referred, had revealed a litany of violence, abuse, and corruption, much of which was connected to the managing role of the penitentiary commissioners. By comparing the commissioners of the temporary asylum to commissioners of the penitentiary, Park not only held them ultimately responsible for similar abuses but also questioned the very role of the commissioner as traditionally defined. Park condemned the asylum commissioners for maintaining and increasing their power by the strategic dispensation of patronage. He referred to the commissioners as aristocrats, members of a provincial elite immune from responsibility to the state who jealously guarded their position of power to the detriment of the asylum. He made direct links between the commissioners' success in awarding asylum contracts to friends and relatives and the poor quality or lack of food and clothing for patients.[36] He considered the retention of asylum employees who were in various ways useful to the commissioners to be damaging to the good order of the asylum and to the effective treatment of patients. Imbued with a sense of the importance of the asylum derived from his reading of European alientists Pinel, Esquirol and Samuel Tuke, founder of the famous York Retreat in England, Park was undoubtedly destined for conflict with the Board of Commissioners.

The opening of the permanent Toronto Provincial Asylum in 1850, ushered in a period in which relations between commissioners and superintendents had a dramatically different character, first with John Scott as superintendent and then under his successor, Joseph Workman. In the period of changeover from the temporary to the permanent asylum, calls were issued from several sources for the creation of a new and better board of commissioners. With the appointment of John Scott (son-in-law of Commissioner Roaf), however, it appeared that the "old machinery" of inspection and administration was reinstituted into the new asylum.[37] But even this seemingly complicit relationship between superintendent and commissioners soon broke down – for reasons quite unlike those that had previously caused discord at the temporary asylum.

Soon after his appointment, Superintendent Scott ran into difficulties with an attendant, John Coppins, who resigned from service over Scott's refusal to let him leave work early to be with his dying child. With his resignation, Coppins left a scathing critique of Scott emphasizing the superintendent's constant abuse of asylum patients and attendants. The asylum commissioners responded to these complaints by cautioning the superintendent but they dismissed the seriousness of the attendant's charges. The matter was revived, however, by W.H. Boulton, a member of the opposition in the Reform government, who raised the motion that Coppins' complaints and other irregularities at the asylum warranted a government inquiry into the superintendent's conduct.[38] Boulton's motion was defeated, and the Reform government was spared the unpleasant prospect of an inquiry potentially critical of the superintendent and the commissioners.

This debacle was followed by an incident that implicated the superintendent in a serious scandal involving the dissection of patients. The issue came to light when the coffin of a patient was investigated at the burial ground and found to contain only a portion of the deceased. This unfortunate episode led to an inquest in which Scott admitted that dead patients' parts were occasionally removed for "anatomical purposes." At the ensuing meeting of the Board of Commissioners, four commissioners voted in favour of Scott's immediate dismissal from office. Despite this clear indication of dissension among board members, the powerful influence of Commissioner Roaf swayed the Board to only reprimand the superintendent strongly without calling for his dismissal.

The commissioners' response to this latest round of difficulties with the asylum superintendent finally pushed the government to reconsider the relationship between the state, the Board of Commissioners, and the asylum. On 11 June 1853 a bill introduced by Reform MPP Dr John Rolf "for the better management of the Provincial Lunatic Asylum" became law. As Thomas Brown points out, the new law was designed to "reduce drastically the power and autonomy of the Board of Commissioners and to place control of the asylum in the hands of the government." To that end, the government replaced the twelve-member permanent, unsalaried board with a visiting four-member board. It also more clearly defined the board's function, empowering it to report on "the manner in which the Institution is conducted," and to "frame such By-laws as may seem to be advisable for the peace, welfare, and good government of the Institution."[39] With the impending dissolution of the old Board of Commissioners, Scott was about to lose his powerful support in the face of increasing hostility to his superintendency. He resigned from office just before the final reading of the new act.

With the appointment of Joseph Workman as Scott's interim replacement, the dynamics between commissioners and superintendent shifted considerably. Unlike Rees, Telfer, and Park, Workman was able to force into place an asylum environment that more closely approximated the medical conception of the ideal asylum. Workman's successes were facilitated by the new Act for the Better Management of the Provincial Lunatic Asylum at Toronto, which changed relationships between asylum officers to permit shaping the asylum into a more "ideal" state institution. However, the long-standing conflicts between the superintendent and the commissioners – and later with asylum inspectors – did not completely come to an end, and emerging conflicts still hinged primarily on differing conceptions of the role of the lunatic asylum as a state institution.

When Workman was appointed permanent superintendent in 1853, the earlier rules and regulations, or bylaws, of the asylum were expanded and modified in ways that would have an important effect on the subsequent working of the institution. The superintendent finally acquired the power to hire and dismiss asylum attendants and servants – a power that previous superintendents had unsuccessfully attempted to wrest away from the commissioners – thereby substantially increasing his influence in the asylum. The position of bursar was created to serve the function of asylum "store keeper," purchasing and supervising all provisions for the institution. The existence of this role reduced the responsibility and power of the steward in the sphere of asylum provisions. A new rule that "no purchases [should] be made from any commissioners, officers or servant of the institution" indicated a clear effort to curtail the tendering-out of contracts through commissioners and other officers at the expense of the asylum. Finally, both the steward and the matron were to ensure that no food or provisions other than were necessary made their way into the hands of the attendants or servants.[40]

Workman had a vision of the asylum consistent with that of Rees, Telfer, and Park. But he was able to use the reconstituted asylum bylaws to his advantage in carrying out a dramatic period of institutional reform. Despite his own set of conflicts with the Board of Commissioners and later with the Board of Inspectors of Asylums, Prisons and Public Charities created in 1858, Workman also managed to retain his position at the asylum for a considerable period, an achievement that enabled him to effect long-term change within the asylum.

In 1854 Workman notified the Board of Commissioners that with the assistance of his new steward he had "discovered that a deeply rooted and ... long continued system of pillage" had existed in the asylum. He was happy, he said, to inform the commissioners that he had uncovered and suppressed this "gross abuse," but the "completeness and disciplined experience of the organization" made it impossible to single out those against whom criminal proceedings could be laid.[41] According to Workman, the purging of this illicit activity began with the sudden retirement of the steward and matron shortly after he had taken up permanent residence at the asylum. He made implicit judgments on both former officials by heralding their replacement by two persons "of established integrity, and of active and well regulated minds."[42]

A short while after moving into the asylum, Workman was struck by the inordinately unhealthy physical and psychological condition of the asylum patients. He decided to investigate whether the diet of the patients was in part responsible for the "depressed, attenuated, and half lifeless state in which they languished." Workman had first suspected something wrong with the food supply in the asylum when, upon arrival, he was sent up "a liberal supply" of butter from the asylum dairy. After inquiries to the "dairy woman," he found that it was customary for the superintendent and steward to receive fresh butter daily from the dairy. Upon further investigation he discovered that out of a total of 47 quarts of milk produced each day by the asylum dairy, 6 quarts were distributed among the 360 patients, 8 quarts were distributed to the 50 employees, and the remaining 33 quarts went unaccounted for either within or outside the asylum. Shortly thereafter the dairy woman retired from the asylum. The superintendent then prohibited the churning of milk into butter, ordered the purchase of better milk cows, and arranged strict supervision of milk production and distribution. Within a short period, 80 to 100 quarts of milk were distributed daily among the patients, and Workman reported a dramatic improvement in patient health.[43]

The new superintendent found similar problems in the distribution of bread and meat in the asylum. He discovered that one of the cooks, who had been a long-time employee of the asylum, was stealing ten to twenty loaves of bread a day. The cook was dismissed immediately, and the quantity of bread available for patients dramatically increased. Workman also estimated that an increase of about 1,000 pounds of meat per month followed the retirement of the late steward.

Still uncertain whether the network of pilferage in the asylum had been fully dealt with, Workman took the extraordinary measure of "closing the channels of exit" of asylum supplies by forbidding all asylum employees from leaving the institution property for the entire month of August. At the end of the month, Workman declared that he had an accurate understanding of the "legitimate consumption of the house in every item of supply." He also was satisfied that the outside connections to the system of institutional theft had been effectively severed.

Workman next set out to purge the institution of employees he considered unworthy of their posts. Making use of the superintendent's newly granted powers of dismissal, he informed the female attendants of an entire ward (in charge of sixty-six patients) that their services would be dispensed with at the end of the month as a result of their general "insubordination and negligence." In an act of protest, the attendants declared their intention to quit immediately and demanded the remainder of their pay. Workman called in the police, who issued a warrant for the nurses' arrest – presumably for illegally breaking their contracts. Faced with this police coercion, the attendants complied with the order to return to their work until their dismissal at the end of the month. Within an hour of this incident, fourteen other female attendants notified Workman that they would resign at the end of the month.[44] The dismissed employees and those who resigned were, in the superintendent's opinion, part of the "formidable corroboration" responsible for the systematic embezzlement of asylum provisions.

Workman's success in bringing the character of the asylum more in line with his vision of a proper state institution marked an important turning point in the history of the state asylum in Ontario. As Charles Rosenberg has pointed out for the American context, early and middle nineteenth-century medical institutions were governed in keeping with the social relations of the society in which they were built.[45] In a period of strict class distinctions, commissioners certainly assumed that all asylum officers, from the superintendent to the servant, were subject to their ultimate authority. But there was also an understanding of reciprocal responsibility between social classes that played out in a complex system of patronage based on close relations between the activities of commissioners and subordinate asylum officers. In this institutional context, asylum attendants and servants saw the perquisites attendant to such patronage – both officially and unofficially sanctioned – as an essential supplement to their subsistence wages.[46] Superintendents, however, with their unique combination of medical and middle-class backgrounds, saw the asylum first and foremost as an institution of therapeutic and moral regulation. During the Workman era, the actual conditions within the institution became more closely aligned with the superintendent's vision of the ideal asylum. This does not mean that the asylum completely embodied the superintendent's ideal of an institution of medical and social control.[47] Nor had the older form of struggle between superintendent and commissioners come to an end.[48] As Workman slowly eradicated those qualities of the asylum that had characterised it as a traditional state institution, new forms of conflict came to the fore between the medical director and the asylum's inspectors.

Once Workman had established good order in his asylum, his appeals to the government and to the commissioners began to focus on overcrowding in the asylum, and this issue soon formed the basis of a renewed round of conflicts between the superintendent and asylum inspectors. On many occasions, Workman had pointed out to the commissioners the overcrowded state of the institution, and he argued that, with a patient population far in excess of its acceptable capacity, the asylum was dangerous. He reminded the commissioners that the two wings originally included in the architectural plans for the asylum had not yet been built.[49] The result was that "neither the mental nor the bodily health of the patients [could] be expected to improve as under more favourable circumstances they would do: consequently the institution must become comparatively inoperative for the great and humane purpose for which ... it [had] been established." In fact Workman argued that the Toronto Asylum was becoming more of a giant house of refuge, a "convenient national poor house," than an institution for the cure of insanity. He therefore suggested that he be given discretion in limiting future admissions so that he might try to re-establish the proper functioning (as he saw it) of the lunatic asylum.[50]

The overcrowding was partially relieved by the establishment of "branch asylums" at the University of Toronto in 1856, at Fort Malden, Amherstburg, in 1859, and at Orillia in 1861.[51] These makeshift institutions were originally intended to take on contingents of "incurables" from the Toronto Asylum who, it was assumed, could be cared for in more modest asylum settings. In theory, the transfer of incurables to the branch asylums would allow Workman to concentrate on curing patients whose illnesses were more recent. This strategy of branch institutions was accompanied in 1856 by a new institutional bylaw granting Workman the powers he had long asked for to "make discrimination in admissions, giving preference to recent acute cases of insanity, over those of long standing." This right to screen admissions was of particular interest to Workman as standard wisdom among alienists of the time was that early detection and treatment of insanity offered patients the best chances of recovery.[52]

Despite the establishment of the branch asylums and Workman's discretionary power over admissions to the Toronto Asylum, a growing demand for admissions made reduction in overcrowding impossible. Although Workman used his "best judgement in awarding vacancies to the most urgent cases," the "arrearage" of applications to the Toronto Asylum grew at an alarming rate.[53] Workman attributed this inexorable demand to two factors. First, the new bylaw giving Workman discretion in admission also stressed the superintendent's responsibility to pay particular attention to admitting "violent or dangerous" patients. This meant in effect that Workman was obliged to give priority of place to those considered insane who were being held in local county jails. Theirs were not always the most recent of cases, nor were their medical problems necessarily the most amenable to asylum therapeutics. Many, he claimed, were in fact paupers, "imbeciles and idiots," or just old and worn out, no longer wanted by their families. Second, although the branch asylums had been built to relieve the burden of the demand for admissions, Workman argued that the number of requests was simply increasing beyond the capacity of these makeshift institutions. What was really needed was the creation of more "purpose built" asylum accommodation for the treatment of "real" lunatics.

On this issue, the views of the superintendent were supported by the asylum commissioners and the newly created Board of Inspectors of Prisons, Asylums and Public Charities.[54] The commissioners had on several occasions endorsed Workman's reports to the government about the dangers of overcrowding. The Board of Inspectors of Asylums also concurred with the superintendent that the scale of accommodation for the insane needed to be radically expanded to meet the ever-increasing demand.[55] Arguing along the same lines as Workman, they claimed that in both Ontario and Quebec inadequate provision for the insane had in fact multiplied the number of incurables. "The extent to which ... the incurables are multiplied can be easily understood, when it is remembered that in the earlier stages of insanity the percentage of curable cases is about 70 or 75%, whereas if from want of asylum accommodation, the patients cannot be brought under treatment for some months after the commencement of the attack, the rate of cures is reduced to 25 or 30%. Thus by delaying the treatment we increase by 50% or one half of the whole number of the insane, the percentage of incurables who are thrown permanently as a burthen on the state."[56] The inspectors fully endorsed Workman's calls for the completion of the wings of the Toronto Asylum, adding their own call for the construction of additional asylums in both provinces.[57]

Despite their concurrence on the issue of overcrowding, however, the asylum inspectors and superintendents remained at odds on the practicalities of admission. A series of apparently minor conflicts over the process of patient committal at the local level highlights their discord. In one instance, the deputy clerk of the United Counties of Lanark and Renfrew alerted the government to a grand jury report that complained that five "lunatics" had been retained in the Perth County jail. One had been imprisoned for five years, another for three years, two others for over two years, and the last for a year and two months. The grand jury put forth the familiar argument that the prolonged presence of these lunatics was disturbing the good order of the prison. The jurors were dismayed to learn that warrants for committal for all five insane prisoners had long ago been sent by the Perth sheriff both to Joseph Workman at the Toronto Asylum and to John Litchfield at the Rockwood Criminal Lunatic Asylum in Kingston, apparently to no avail. The grand jury's complaint prompted the provincial government to sanction the removal of four of the patients to the Toronto Asylum if the superintendent found room to accommodate them.[58]

Workman responded by reminding the government of the asylum bylaw authorizing him to admit patients selectively according to the recency and nature of their insanity. He strongly reiterated his argument that exercise of this discretion was the only means of keeping the asylum functioning as a curative institution rather than a refuge for all manner of society's outcasts. In his opinion the four lunatics in question at the Perth jail were "confirmed incurables" for whom accommodation at the Toronto Asylum would be of no benefit whatsoever. This, the superintendent informed the government, he had made quite clear to the sheriff of Perth. He made the accusation that the Perth officials' persistence in seeking warrants for their removal to an asylum reflected "municipal financial considerations," and not a concern for the acute or violent nature of the insanity of the lunatics confined in the jail. Workman noted that the practice of issuing warrants for the removal of harmless and incurable lunatics from local jails was common and frequently led to the committal of insane patients to the asylum who, in his view, should never have been sent there. Such individuals, Workman argued, ought to be cared for at home by family or friends. On the basis of these arguments, he withheld his approval for admission of the lunatics from the Perth Jail.[59]

Workman's response to the government did not close the debate, however. The provincial secretary next called on the asylum inspectors to investigate and report on the affair. Inspector Taché, chairman of the Board of Inspectors, reported that he was in one sense sympathetic to Workman's efforts to make the Toronto Asylum "a corrective institution rather than a mere Boarding House for the incurable insane." He argued, however, that "as an Inspector" he believed there were other considerations and responsibilities that prevented him from concurring with the decision of the superintendent.

To take care of the insane, is a duty of the State, that relates as well to the incurable Lunatics and Idiots, as to the curable: the degree of comfort to be allowed to those unfortunate beings, must necessarily be measured by the means of the State called upon to receive them in its Public Institutions. In accordance with those premises, I say that we are bound to receive the insane in our asylums, and that our asylum accommodations not being quite adequate to the wants, are, by necessity, obliged to crowd these institutions as much as they can be without incurring an immediate danger for the general health of their inmates.[60]

Although sympathetic to Workman's vision of the asylum as a well-ordered institution for the cure of insanity, the inspectors thought that the therapeutic function of the asylum should not take precedence over the state's responsibility to provide accommodation for incurables and idiots as well as for those whose insanity showed promise of cure. Had they been put into effect, Taché's ideas would have led to the creation of the very kind of receptacle for the maintenance of incurables that the superintendent had vigorously opposed.

When the provincial secretary forwarded Inspector Taché's recommendation that the state be responsible for the admission of the Perth lunatics to the Toronto Asylum, Workman was obliged to comply. He reported that although he hoped "His Excellency does not suppose that I concur in Dr Taché's views," the Perth inmates had, as requested, been sent to asylums: one to the Toronto Asylum and the others to the Rockwood Asylum. To further emphasize his disapproval of asylum inspector's decision, Workman observed that the patient sent to the Toronto Asylum showed no signs of insanity. She was "constantly industrious, quiet, and totally inoffensive ... by no means, one of those [cases] which I regard as having preferential claim to the benefits of this asylum."[61]

The battle over the committal of the Perth lunatics suggests that the attitudes of the inspectors and medical superintendents were not the only forces at work in shaping the Toronto Asylum. Debate over the appropriate role for the asylum was heated at the municipal and county level also and had an important impact on the use and character of the state institution. Concerns expressed at the local level often conflicted with both asylum superintendent and state inspectors.

As the example of Perth demonstrates, much of the pressure for increased accommodation at the Toronto and branch asylums emanated from local communities. From the point of view of the local district jail, the local justice of the peace, the district grand jury, and, of course, individual families, the main concern was to acquire admittance for those considered insane (or otherwise undesirable) to the new public institution which had been established for the purpose of housing them. Since the insane were often seen as a burden to individual families and to the community and as a disruption to the discipline and order of many district jails, delays in acquiring asylum committal resulted in complaints at the community level.

The municipal council of the united counties of Huron and Bruce complained that "lunatics [had] been at different times confined in the jail of these counties until a vacancy occurred in the asylum." The council argued that its local jail had neither the "appliances" nor the expertise to properly treat the insane, and noted that, as the province's population was rapidly growing, the need for increased accommodation for the insane was becoming ever more acute. The municipal council of Wellington lodged a similar complaint: "It is quite impossible to secure the admission of a lunatic ... short of two or three months, however deep seated or violent the demeanour of the patient." The Waterloo municipal council, in its appeal for more asylum space, emphasized the disruption that the presence of the insane caused to the debtors and criminal offenders of their prison.[62]

In their efforts to push the state to increase provision for the insane, some counties made selective use of the arguments of superintendents and asylum inspectors. Referring to the printed annual reports of the medical superintendent of the Toronto Asylum, the surgeon of the Norfolk County jail, John Clarke, repeated the theory that the longer the delay in getting patients from the jail to the asylum the greater the chance of their insanity being impossible to treat and that delays in committal due to lack of provision thus increased the numbers of the incurably insane. However, adopting the argument of asylum inspectors, Clarke also urged provision of more asylum accommodation for the incurably insane, whose treatment in a properly ordered asylum would be far more humane than in the local prison.[63]

Such complaints from all around Ontario increased the pressure for Workman to accommodate the insane from local jails in accordance with the intent of the 1856 asylum bylaw. But as many of the locally confined patients had conditions that Workman considered untreatable, they were in his mind ineligible for the Toronto Asylum. Moreover, Workman frequently accused local communities of purposefully incarcerating people judged to be insane in local jails regardless of whether they were violent or dangerous (or, for that matter, actually insane) in order to secure for them a "preferential consideration" for removal to the asylum. In his opinion "it would be indiscrete and unjust, to place the beds of this institution preferentially at command of applicants seeking admission in this way."[64]

To emphasize his point, Workman recounted the case of Mary Murray, an alleged lunatic who had received a warrant for admission to the Toronto Asylum while incarcerated in the Barrie local jail. Workman had her sent down to the asylum. Upon examining her documents, he discovered that her medical certificates of insanity had been made out not by doctors in Barrie but by three doctors in Toronto. Workman concluded that in filling out their certificates the Toronto physicians had relied on information given by the official in charge of transporting Murray to the asylum. The physicians who filled out the certificates of insanity that made Murray's admission to the asylum legal had no knowledge of her medical history. Workman could not find any indication that she was insane. In the course of several discussions with Murray, Workman learned that she had an abusive husband who had committed her to the Barrie local jail under charges of being insane and dangerous to be at large. The superintendent decided to keep Murray at the asylum until the spring, as she appeared to him to be physically weak and unable to withstand the winter weather. He argued that Murray's case was characteristic of a large number of patients sent from the province's county jails.[65] In sending patients like Murray to the Toronto Asylum, local communities were bound for conflict with a superintendent committed to restricting his institution to the treatment and cure of medically and scientifically "legitimate" lunatics.

In an effort to mediate the conflicts arising between the superintendent and the communities, the state issued a circular to all the province's counties ordering them to provide a list of all insane persons committed to the local jails, the dates of committal, and the offences or other reasons for their incarceration. The counties were also ordered to inform the government immediately of any subsequent non-criminal admissions the local jails and to provide the same information for them. In this way the state hoped to keep track of the numbers of mentally ill being incarcerated at the local level and also to gain some idea of those whose cases merited early committal to the lunatic asylum. The response to these circulars indicated to the government that many people were being committed to local jails as insane. They were alleged to have committed crimes of assault or petty theft, or considered dangerous to be at large.[66] In the eyes of community members, the reports from the local jails served to highlight the need for increased accommodation for those considered to be insane.

Community frustration over the difficulty of getting the mentally ill moved quickly from the local jail to the state asylum was linked to conflicts over the state asylum tax. As early as 1843 the councillors of the Niagara District, for example, had argued that although the community had been taxed the heavy sum of £1,104.6.6 since 1839 for the erection of a permanent lunatic asylum, the construction of that asylum had not yet begun. This tax was in addition to the annual £407 levied for the maintenance of the insane within the district. The councillors were also frustrated because the temporary asylum seemed to them "to be principally beneficial to the Home District although supported by Provincial funds." A similar petition from the municipal council of the District of Newcastle noted: "There is a general impression throughout the province that a sum sufficiently ample to meet the expense [for the erection of a permanent asylum] has already been raised, and paid into the hands of the Receiver General." Other petitions urged the immediate application of the asylum tax to asylum construction in order to relieve the insane of the "cruel sufferings" that resulted from their wandering about at large and from their incarceration in the local jails.[67]

The animosity of counties and municipalities towards the state asylum tax was not abated by the eventual opening of the permanent Toronto Provincial Asylum in 1850. After 1850 the state asylum tax was replaced by an asylum fund tax that was to help pay for the maintenance, renovations and additions to the asylum. Nevertheless the asylum continued to be hampered by ongoing financial difficulties, and in 1852 the commissioners decided temporarily to accept only patients who could pay the weekly expenses of asylum accommodation. This restriction aroused immediate outrage at the local level. As the warden of the Hastings County jail informed the provincial secretary: "This county pays about £300 a year towards the asylum fund and we certainly do not expect to pay such an annual contribution, and then be told that because an insane person belongs to a poor family ... he can find no aid, no relief in an asylum thus munificently supported." Members of the municipal council of Lincoln and Welland Counties expressed the same objection, adding that the "enormous sums annually collected for the liquidation of the debt" on asylum buildings should easily cover the costs of managing the institution. They petitioned the government to reduce the asylum tax and to make an inquiry into the "abuses which seem to obtain in the monetary affairs of that charity."[68]

Some local petitions made an explicit connection between appeals for expanded asylum accommodation and the multiple burdens of taxation. Petitioners complained that as well as paying the asylum fund tax levied by the government they were forced to pay for the medical treatment and general maintenance in the local jails of the mentally ill for whom asylum accommodation could not be provided. Moreover, some counties noted that the annual monies that they submitted for the maintenance of the insane were far in excess of the amount required to maintain patients from their areas in the Toronto Asylum.[69] Such complaints about the asylum tax were ignored by government officials.

The study of community attitudes about the proper role of the state lunatic asylum and an analysis of the struggles between the community, the medical superintendent and government officials are essential to an understanding of the development of the asylum in Ontario. Although the "idea" of the state lunatic asylum and its intended ideological function was grounded firmly in the social thought of middle-class alienists and asylum proponents, the actual development of the asylum as a state institution was more influenced by the competing visions of various class and political groupings in nineteenth-century Ontario. During the era of the temporary, or provisional, asylum, clashes between asylum commissioners and superintendents highlighted differences between elitist perceptions of the public institution as an arena for the exercise of patronage, privilege, and status, and a vision of the asylum as a space in which the social and medical cure and control of madness would best be achieved. Once the permanent Toronto Asylum and its subsequent branch institutions had been established, the conceptions of asylum inspectors and superintendents, though more consistent in some respects, still differed in crucial ways. The resulting conflicts fundamentally affected the development of the institutional response to insanity in Ontario. Further working against asylum superintendents' realization of the ideal lunatic asylum was the committal of patients from the community who were not, in their view, genuine lunatics in need of asylum therapy. The resulting compromises indicated the extent to which community and state perceptions of the asylum's purpose and significance played an influential role in shaping the character of state provision for the insane.

3 Medicine, Moral Therapy, and Madness in Nineteenth-Century Quebec and Ontario

The study of moral treatment and its institutional expression, the lunatic asylum, has been of central importance to historians of nineteenth-century psychiatry. In an ongoing historiographical debate, historians, historical sociologists, philosophers, and historically minded psychiatrists have argued over the significance of the conjuncture of asylum development, moral treatment, and the professionalization of psychiatry.[1] The focus of most of these histories has been the rise and development of the asylum and asylum medicine, while other socio-medical means of treatment of the insane have been neglected. In works where pre- and non-asylum forms of medical treatment and diagnosis of insanity are acknowledged, historians have ceased looking for them after the establishment of the asylum.[2] One partial exception can be found in the work of Nancy Tomes. In an analysis of correspondence between patrons of the Pennsylvania Hospital for the Insane and its Superintendent, Thomas Kirkbride, Tomes has uncovered a wealth of information on "patrons' conceptions of insanity and its causes; the circumstances leading to commitment, including prior treatment; and the dynamics of the doctor-patron relationship." Tomes argues that Kirkbride, "within the intellectual and practical bounds of his medical training, ... chose a therapeutic method that appealed to his lay clientele," and that a "shared consensus regarding the origins and treatment of mental disorders" emerged between asylum superintendents and asylum patrons at the hospital.[3]

This aspect of Tomes's work serves as a point of departure, for a broader investigation of the history of medicine, therapy, and insanity in nineteenth-century Ontario and Quebec without diminishing the importance of the development of the asylum and of the medical theory and practice emanating from it.[4] Although a large proportion of those considered insane in both provinces were treated in lunatic asylums, medicine and therapy were also practised in socio-medical contexts beyond these institutions. Medical evaluations and treatments did not begin upon patients' arrival at the asylum door but well before their committal to an asylum. Moreover, as the previous two chapters have shown, asylum accommodation in both provinces was considered by alienists and government officials to be inadequate to accommodate all who were perceived to be insane. There were by some accounts as many alleged lunatics "at large" as there were under institutional treatment.[5] How were people whose insanity did not result in a trip to the asylum diagnosed and treated?

In an insightful article, historian Patricia Prestwich describes the common situation: "Families had integrated the asylum into their own well-established systems of treatment for the mentally disturbed or chronically ill, systems that made skillful use of various formal and informal resources available in the family, neighborhood, and the larger community. When these resources failed, they turned to the asylum, but not necessarily as a permanent or longterm alternative."[6] This chapter points out and analyzes in greater detail some of those formal and informal family and community resources and their relationship to lunatic asylums as these new "curative institutions" became more commonplace over the course of the nineteenth century.[7]

In Ontario and Quebec, there were a variety of integrally connected socio-medical contexts – including the provisional asylum, permanent asylum, local jail, general hospital, and the local community – in which patients were evaluated and treated as insane. The temporary asylum era in Ontario saw an interesting transitional phase in therapeutics from an essentially "heroic" system of treatment of the insane to one more oriented toward "moral therapy." In both provinces, medicine and therapy were constrained by the buildings in which the temporary asylums were housed.

The permanent asylums ushered in an era of moral therapy proper; however, treatment in them could only approximate the ideals of their medical superintendents. Despite their emergence in both provinces at mid-century, the permanent asylums failed to reduce the numbers of insane held in the local jails of Ontario and Quebec. In fact local jails continued to receive and accommodate the insane for prolonged periods. In many jails, physicians or surgeons were hired for the purpose of tending to the needs of the inmates, among whom were some mentally ill patients. In some instances distinct systems of treatment and care of the insane developed in local jails. The jail evolved into a social and medical gateway between the community and the asylum through which local concerns and perceptions were translated into requests for institutional committal and treatment. In Quebec, a variety of institutions, including the *système des loges* in the cities of Montreal, Quebec, and Trois Rivières and in various charitable hospitals in the province, also served as medical and therapeutic settings for the insane. Medical practices of local physicians further contributed to the complex matrix of medicine, therapy, and insanity. Finally, families' and friends' perceptions of insanity were fundamental in the initial diagnosis and treatment of those they considered to be insane.

The introduction of the lunatic asylum had a significant effect on the nature of medicine, therapy, and the treatment of insanity in Ontario and Quebec. The earlier socio-medical contexts in which the insane had been evaluated and treated did not disappear with the rise of the asylum, however. The asylum became integrated into a complex pre-existing network of medical and therapeutic responses to insanity. To the extent that asylum doctors acknowledged the various components of this network of non-asylum forms of medical and therapeutic intervention, they decried their existence and blamed the relative ineffectiveness of asylum treatment on their perpetuation. In both provinces, tension and conflict more often than consensus characterized relations between asylum physicians and officials and their counterparts in communities.[8] This tension suggests that in nineteenth-century Canada, there was relatively little medicalization "from above" of lay ideas about insanity and the "appropriate" use of the lunatic asylum.[9] It is reasonable to presume that the asylum and psychiatric medicine did to some extent come to affect local lay and medical conceptualizations of insanity, but the asylum was not cultivated on unbroken therapeutic ground. As new forms of treatment of insanity developed over the course of the century, the asylum itself was equally influenced by pre-existing mechanisms for dealing with the insane and by the social and therapeutic attitudes that they represented.

In Ontario and Quebec provisional asylums for the insane were established at about the same time: in Montreal on 1 November 1839, and in Toronto on 21 January 1841. Both institutions were located in spaces formerly used as jails – the Toronto Temporary Asylum was established in the abandoned Home District Jail, and the Montreal Lunatic Asylum occupied the third floor of the Montreal District Jail. In both cases the respective governments had intended these institutions to be only temporary responses to the need for institutional accommodation of the insane. They were to have been quickly replaced by permanent purpose-built accommodation. Both provisional institutions operated for longer than anticipated, however, the Montreal asylum for about five years, the Toronto asylum for ten.

What primary documentation exists for the Montreal Temporary Asylum indicates that its treatment was essentially non-somatic with elements of moral treatment in evidence. Although that facility was opened in the fall of 1839, its physician, Dr Jean-Baptiste-Curtius Trestler, was not appointed to the asylum until May 1841.[10] The rules and regulations for the asylum suggest that a tight daily regimen was considered an important part of patient therapy.[11] There are also indications that a limited range of work-related activities were encouraged and carried out on an airing ground, designed to provide daily exercise for patients.[12] Cold showers, straight jackets, and isolation were employed for refractory patients; however, attendants or keepers were instructed to address patients with "a mild and gentle tone of voice" and, in response to patient abuse and unrest, to "keep cool, forbear to recriminate, to scold, threaten or dictate in the language of authority."[13] This attitude towards patients was certainly in keeping with theoretical models of nineteenth-century moral treatment. The third floor of the jail had been renovated to provide a male and a female ward, each with eight patient rooms measuring 12 feet by 9 feet.[14] As early as 1843 two to three patients were crowded into

each room, a situation that Trestler complained "strongly militated against the success of ... their treatment."[15] Despite the overcrowded state of the temporary asylum and other incidents that
appeared to disrupt effective medical treatment, the institution's
officers claimed a high success rate. Between 1839 and 1844 the
Montreal asylum treated 196 patients of whom 98 were released
as cured and 25 were described as "improved."[16]

Early medicine and therapy at the Toronto Temporary Asylum
contrasted in several important ways with therapeutic practices at
its institutional counterpart in Montreal. From 1840 to 1844 the
Toronto temporary asylum's first alienist, Dr William Rees, relied
heavily on "antiphlogistic" or "depletive therapy" in his medical
practice. According to this theory, cure was best achieved through
"the exclusion and removal of all external causes of irritation, and
in reducing and tranquillizing inordinate action of the vascular
nervous and voluntary systems, by the most energetic means, local
and general and by attention to regulation of the animal function."[17] This "counter-irritation" therapy was an effort to restore
the physiological balance of the patient, which had been disturbed
with the onset of mental alienation. Rees's antiphlogistic treatment
included bleeding, cupping, the application of blisters of Spanish
flies, and the use of setons to remove amounts of blood appropriate to the patient's condition. Nauseating doses of antimony and
tartar emetic were used as purgatives. Rees also employed cold
"affusion" on the shaved head and low diet in his treatment.[18]

Although Rees's active depletion therapy was a debated medical
issue by the 1840s, some physicians of insanity still considered it to
be appropriate treatment for certain recent cases of mental aberration. Much more controversial, however, was his use of this aggressive antiphlogistic treatment for patients whose insanity was
long-term, who constituted a majority at the temporary asylum.
According to Rees, antiphlogistic therapy through the use of blisters and setons arrested the progress of the disease in incurable
cases, thereby relieving the asylum of "any of the painful cases of
the loss of the voluntary powers, which would render them a burden intolerable, both to themselves and to the institution, during
the remainder of their lives."[19]

Rees justified his aggressive therapeutic strategy on medical
grounds. By the end of his career at the temporary lunatic asylum, he boasted a patient cure rate of 60 per cent, as high as that

of many lunatic asylums in Europe or the United States. But his interventionist approach was also in part necessitated by the constraints that the architecture of the temporary asylum placed on his ability to pursue moral treatment. Rees frequently complained of the overcrowded state of the institution and his resulting inability to provide proper work, exercise, and amusements to help the recovery of his patients. He also lamented the impossibility of effecting a classification of patients beyond the simple separation of male from female patients and the refractory from the quiet. In the absence of the means for moral therapy, depletive therapy was, he argued, the best medical treatment for his patients.

Yet it is unlikely that Rees would have wholly abandoned his depletive therapy – and the medical outlook into which it fit – even if the temporary asylum had been more amenable to moral treatment. He was, in fact, an interesting transitional figure in alienist therapeutics, who had absorbed an eclectic mix of heroic and moral approaches to the treatment of the insane. Following the lead of the prominent European alienists François Broussais and J.C. Pritchard, Rees was still convinced that many chronic forms of mania could be improved or held in check by the use of counter-irritation.[20] And, in keeping with the medical writings of Benjamin Rush, Achille Foville, Broussais and others, he saw newly contracted cases of mania as inflammatory diseases that would respond positively to aggressive depletive therapy.[21] But at the same time Rees was one of Upper Canada's early proponents of the establishment of a state lunatic asylum, an institution in which the architecture and the internal and external organization embodied the main principles of moral treatment advocated by alienists Philipe Pinel, Samuel and Daniel Tuke, and their substantial group of followers. Rees continually complained that in the absence of moral therapeutic components the recovery of his patients, especially convalescent patients who had responded favourably to his antiphlogistic therapy, was inhibited. Also in keeping with the principles of moral treatment, Rees prohibited the use of mechanical restraint during his superintendency.

Towards the end of his career, Rees's asylum therapeutics came under fire from some of the physician commissioners of the temporary asylum, one of whom, Dr Telfer, became Rees's successor as superintendent. The criticisms of Rees's aggressive somatic approach were linked in part to the broader conflicts between commissioners and superintendents at the asylum. But they also indicated a growing distrust of antiphlogistic therapeutics, which had in most parts of Europe and North America been eclipsed by the philosophy and medical practice of moral treatment.

Rees's retirement after sustaining a serious injury from a blow on the head by one of his patients marked an abrupt end to depletive therapy at the temporary asylum. Rees's three successors, Superintendents Telfer, Park, and Primrose, had similar approaches to the medical treatment of the insane. In contrast to Rees, however, they advocated a combination of treatments that included opiates to procure sleep, a generous diet, and the regulation of the bowels in acute cases of insanity. Chronic patients were given stimulants such as wine, beer, and brandy in order to "induce greater action of the heart, thereby giving a more healthy action to the brain." In chronic cases, a full diet was also considered to improve the "mental faculties."[22]

Telfer, Park, and Primrose tried to combine this less obtrusive medical regimen with other recommended practices of moral therapy. Despite their frequent complaints about the physical limitations of the temporary asylum building, they tried to engage patients in various "amusements" such as dancing, singing, reading, draughts, and cards. The superintendents also encouraged patients to work at gender-appropriate tasks. Women were employed in sewing and knitting supplies for the institution, and gardening work was provided for the men after the conversion of the east wing of the parliament building on Front Street West in Toronto to a branch asylum. The branch asylum also increased the scope for patient exercise and open air walks. To round out the practice of moral treatment, religious services were offered at both institutions. In keeping with newly adopted contemporary medical principles, these aspects of moral treatment were considered as important diversions from the morbid associations of the diseased brain. Physical activity was also thought to be an essential stimulant to cerebral function.[23] There was considerable consistency between the medical perspective of the superintendents at the temporary asylums at Toronto and Montreal and those of the first permanent institutions in Ontario and Quebec. But while the alienists of the temporary asylums were forced to compromise their treatment ideals in institutions not designed for the purpose, the permanent asylums offered, in theory at least, the chance for medical therapy to be practised as intended in purpose-built asylums.

The permanent asylum was considered to be the institutional expression of moral treatment and thus was essential to successful therapy. The asylum itself was to be strategically located in an area that would promote the health of the patients, with soothing panoramic views and access to fresh water. Its design was intended to afford the means for the medical classification and segregation of the insane according to gender, mental disease, behaviour, and class background. Although recommendations on the optimal size of the patient population varied, it was considered important not to treat more than 250 patients in one asylum. Built into the asylum's design was the outward and inward appearance of symmetry and orderliness. Architectural symmetry was meant to work in combination with a carefully supervised daily regimen of patient activities to bring about the reordering of disordered minds. Asylum architecture was also supposed to provide the means for work therapy: a large farm was considered essential, as were workshops and knitting and sewing rooms. Moreover, the asylum design was to facilitate a wide range of patient amusements, from daily walks on the asylum grounds to reading from a collection of carefully selected books in the patient library. The living quarters of the superintendent, who had supreme medical and moral power in the institution, were symbolically situated in the centre of the main building at the heart of the institution. Patient attendants and asylum servants were considered vital to moral treatment, and their behaviour towards patients and their superior officers was to match the architectural order of the institution itself.[24]

In Ontario and Quebec as elsewhere, the theory behind the architectural component of moral treatment could not easily be put into practice. Although in both provinces similar problems with the asylum as curative architecture emerged, Quebec more closely approximated the ideal in this aspect of asylum therapeutics, at least until Confederation. According to Joseph Workman, the Toronto Permanent Asylum's first superintendent, not only did the architecture of the Toronto Asylum fail in many ways to enhance the condition of the insane but until about 1856 the institution actually constituted a major health hazard for its patients.

Suspicions about the architectural failings of the Toronto Asylum began after two serious bouts of cholera swept through the institution in 1850 and in 1852.[25] In order to check possible reasons for the severity of the disease among the patients, a sub-committee of the Board of Commissioners was set up to investigate conditions at the asylum. The committee discovered four major problems. First, an examination of the tank on the asylum cupola that supplied water to the institution revealed that a drainage pipe designed to carry off surplus water to prevent its overflow onto the floor was in fact carrying a "noisome effluvia" up to the level of the water tank. Second, an examination of the water closets showed that their construction was flawed they were in a "filthy and pernicious" state. The committee recommended their immediate removal and replacement. Third, the committee reported that the general quality of asylum air was close and foul, a failing that they attributed to the completely ineffective ventilation system of the asylum. Finally, the committee detected in the basement "a very offensive odour arising under the floor of the eastern compartment" that they concluded was produced by the "dirty water from the washing house which passe[d] along an open drain under the floor to the sewer."[26]

These findings prompted more inquiries into the architectural soundness of the asylum. Professor Henry Croft of the University of Toronto was invited to assess the asylum's engineering design. Croft voiced vehement criticism of the asylum, noting that "the system of drainage [was] as unsound in principle as that of ventilation." This report incited a fierce rebuttal from the asylum architect, John Howard, who defended his design and castigated government officials for not completing the asylum wings as originally planned.[27] Shortly after his appointment as medical superintendent of the Toronto Asylum, Workman added his own concerns about the architecture of the new institution. He suspected that frequent outbreaks of epidemic disease and general ill-health in the asylum could be traced to "local causes, connected with the structure and condition of the house."[28] In his subsequent investigations into the relationship between asylum design and patient health, Workman uncovered an environmental disaster.

In searching for the cause of the exceptionally bad quality of the air and drinking water in the asylum, Workman discovered that the distance between the discharge pipe of the "foul contents" of the asylum and the intake pipe that supplied the institution's fresh water from Lake Ontario was only 100 feet. The resulting mix of foul and fresh water pumped back into the institution for patient use was very impure: "Throughout the hot weather [it] has so offensive an odour and taste as to be disagreeable to every patient ... and cannot but be hurtful to their general health." Further investigation led Workman to the discovery of two large cesspools connecting the asylum's water closet drains with the foundation drains. Despite the architect's intention to have these cesspools cleaned out twice yearly, they had not been drained during the three years since the asylum had been opened. Workman feared that "their foul contents may have polluted the basement," causing advanced decay in many of the floorboards and joists. These difficulties only compounded the overriding problem associated with the choice of setting for the asylum. In his view: "It is questionable if a worse site could have been found in the whole province." Far from being in a "salubrious" location conducive to good patient health, the Toronto Asylum grounds were scarcely above the level of the lake, rendering the soil constantly damp. Moreover the low level of the ground interfered with the drainage of the asylum's refuse into the lake. Consequently, "stagnant water, in some places to a considerable depth" was, Workman suspected, frequently detained underneath the asylum.[29]

As as the superintendent grew more familiar with the asylum's patient population, he became convinced that there was a connection between the "type of bodily and mental disease which prevailed throughout the establishment" and the existence of "some prolific source of miasma" in the asylum, beyond what he had yet discovered. He ordered the systematic cleaning and excavation of the drainage system of the asylum. When his investigation reached the level of the basement, the entire foundation of the asylum was found to be flooded with "a mass of filth and impure fluids." The "filth" in the foundation beneath the asylum kitchen measured between 3 and 5 feet in depth. The contamination of the foundation led to extensive timber rot in the basement and upper stories of the asylum. Further search led to the heart of the problem. As Workman reported:

The deep basement drains, leading from the laundries, kitchens and other parts adjacent towards the main sewer, were found to terminate abruptly, at a depth of nine feet, at the south wall of the asylum, under the water closets ... The dirty water of four years, supplied by the kitchens and laundries, had been without any outlet, and having in a very short time, filled and choked the drains, it worked its way up through the soil, and was diffused over a large portion of the entire foundation ... The only disbursing agency, by which it had been kept in check, and prevented from rising above the floors and inundating the whole of the basement, must have been evaporation. Here was a source of morbific agency not merely adequate to destroy the health of the asylum, but even of the neighbourhood.[30]

In their haste to complete the permanent asylum, the architect and contractors had not connected the deep basement drains to the main sewer. Workman estimated that half of the patient deaths in the institution since its opening were attributable to the "pestilent air of the house generated by the filth and decaying timbers of the basement."[31]

Workman's analysis of the effects of the contaminated asylum foundation on the health of his patient population was directly linked to prevailing models of miasmatic disease. He believed, along with many of his contemporaries, that the accumulation of decaying matter, including marshy environments, excreta, and rotting wood, could lead to the contamination of the surrounding air with miasmas. The proliferation of miasmatic air could, in turn, under the right environmental conditions such as a period of intense heat, lead to the spontaneous eruption of epidemic disease or facilitate the spread of such diseases from other sources. Workman attributed the outbreaks of cholera to "local causes connected with the structure and condition of the house" and he feared the spontaneous outbreak of other diseases such as "malignant typhus."[32] The subsequent cleanup of the building foundation further confirmed Workman's assessment of the consequences of the defective asylum architecture. Although he waited until the cool weather of November and December before attempting to remove the miasmatic matter, Workman reported that the asylum matron, several servants, and a few patients were "prostrated by miasmatic fever" upon the removal of the floor boards. More patients suffered when put to work hauling the contaminated soil in buckets and wheelbarrows from the foundation to a distant location.[33]

Workman was convinced that other architectural flaws in the asylum also impaired the physical health and impeded the mental recovery of his patients. Although the cleanup of the foundation had brought a dramatic improvement in the air quality of the asylum, he noted that the institution's ventilation system remained completely defective. This lack of ventilation resulted in the creation of "rarefied air," which, he claimed, was "well known to be depressive of nervous energy and debilitating on muscular power – two physiological results above all others to be averted in the treatment of insanity."[34] He also considered the perpetually overcrowded state of the asylum as "instrumental in depressing the vital powers of the inmates, and ... detract[ing] largely from the curative efficiency of the institution." In his opinion, overcrowding also contributed to the onset of a range of diseases in the institution, including a skin condition called erysipelas, intermittent fevers, and disorders "of the organs of digestion and respiration."[35]

The fact that the asylum wings which had been part of the institution's original design had not yet been built was especially problematic. It was assumed in the theory of moral treatment that they were essential to the proper classification of the various forms and manifestations of mental alienation. Despite the superintendent's repeated explanations of the serious medical consequences of the incompleted plan, the wings were not built until 1867. Workman noted that in most "well ordered" lunatic asylums, such as those in the United States and England at the time, patients were divided into at least nine classes for each sex. Given the architectural limitations at the Toronto Asylum, he was only able to classify his patients into three large divisions.[36] He complained that his inability to separate "the noisy, the violent, the obscene, the epileptic, the filthy, the helpless, the timid and the sick" into their proper wards rendered the asylum "almost useless for curative purposes."[37]

Over the course of the century, the problems of classification and overcrowding were both somewhat relieved with the establishment of branch asylums in the province. The University Branch was opened in 1856, the Malden Branch in 1859, and the Orillia Branch in 1861. These branch asylums were not purpose-built for the cure and treatment of insanity (being a converted university building, fort barrack, and hotel respectively). However, as they were intended to take only contingents of chronically insane or incurable patients sent by Workman from the Toronto Asylum, they were considered architecturally fit institutions for that purpose. The strategy behind these satellite asylums was both economic and therapeutic. The cost of converting them for their new function was lower than the estimate for constructing the wings for the Toronto Asylum. With incurables removed from the Toronto Asylum and new legislation allowing him to be more selective in admitting new patients, Workman was finally in a position to run his asylum as the curative institution it was intended to be. The establishment of the Rockwood Criminal Lunatic Asylum in 1855 was further expected to help Workman's classification and cure of patients.

The promise of these developments for the more efficient practice of moral therapy was, however, compromised by the growing backlog of requests for committal to the asylums and the inevitable overcrowding of the psychiatric institutions. Moreover, there is evidence to suggest that a more ambitious round of state asylum construction later on in the century, with the conversion of Rockwood into an asylum for the "ordinary" insane and the opening of the London Asylum in 1876, tended to reproduce some of the architectural deficiencies of the earlier Toronto institution.[38] But by then, the earlier theoretical relationship between asylum architecture and medical practice was becoming outmoded as new and more pessimistic understandings of insanity and its treatment came to the fore.[39]

Quebec's early asylum architecture came closer than that of Ontario to approximating the theory and practice of moral treatment. Although motivated by profit, Beauport's proprietors were also driven by a sense of professional pride and were informed of the prevailing alienist conceptions of insanity and its proper treatment. In 1845 Drs Douglas, Frémont, and Morrin established what they referred to as a temporary asylum on a property about two and a half miles outside of Quebec City. The 200-acre property contained an old manor house that had been converted into the asylum's main building, capable of accommodating 120 patients.[40] By 1849 Beauport's proprietors had begun construction of a new permanent asylum on a 70-acre property at La Canardière, one and a quarter miles from Quebec, that afforded a good view of the city harbour. The main building was 217 feet long with wings, each measuring 132 feet in length, extending from either side of it. Its design resembled the recommended form for the nineteenth-century lunatic asylum. Plentiful fresh water was supplied by a river on the premises, and the main wash house was located in a building separate from the main asylum.

Patients were divided by gender with male patients occupying the west wing and female patients the east wing. Each group was in turn divided into four principal classifications: the "idiotic" and "intractable or filthy"; patients whose habits were "more orderly"; the quiet; and the convalescent. Within wards there was room for the further subdivision of the patients in each class. The asylum was considered by commissioners and proprietors to afford the "complete means of classification ... a place for exercise and amusement [and] thorough ventilation." Its three proprietors were proud of their facility: "The present Building, as now completed will be found to possess every arrangement which modern experience has taught to be essential to the curative or custodial treatment of the insane."[41]

Despite their overall satisfaction with the architectural features of the asylum, Douglas, Frémont, and Morrin found that their institution was not immune from defects similar to those that plagued the Toronto Asylum. As private entrepreneurs, however, they were not likely to draw the deficiencies of their institution's architecture to the attention of commissioners and state officials. Nor did the peculiar relationship between the state and the Beauport proprietors tend to invite criticism from the government. Nevertheless, there are official indications that the institution's ventilation and heating systems were insufficient to meet the needs of its large patient population.[42] A critical report detailing the conditions at Beauport was produced by the 1887 Royal Commission on Lunatic Asylums of the Province of Quebec. It concluded that the "comfort, health and safety of the patients" were constantly wanting, and that the food and clothing of the patients left much to be desired.[43]

An additional drawback to the Beauport Asylum was that its large size and high population density – neither of which were ideal characteristics according to the theory of architecture as moral therapy – made it vulnerable to fire hazards. On 2 February 1855, a fire destroyed the west wing. Although there were no injuries, the fire caused massive disruption, and the patients were transferred to the Quebec Marine and Emigrant Hospital, where they remained until a new wing was completed at the asylum.[44] In January 1875, a much more devastating fire ripped through the main building at

Beauport killing twenty-six patients and, according to the proprietors, severely aggravating the insane condition of many others.[45] A similar tragedy with an even greater loss of life occurred in Longue Pointe at the St Jean de Dieu Asylum in 1890.[46]

The Beauport proprietors' commitment to "custodial treatment" as well as the cure of the insane marked a therapeutic divergence from their alienist counterparts in Ontario. In fact from the Beauport Asylum's inception, it was acknowledged that a certain percentage of patients classified as incurables would be admitted. Although the Beauport proprietors' willingness to take on this class of patient indicated their major philosophical disagreement with Workman of the Toronto Asylum, the actual reality of medical practices in the two institutions was in many ways the same. Despite Beauport's apparent superiority in design according to the principles of moral treatment, over time both institutions became populated predominantly by patients classified as chronic and incurable. Although officially mandated to accommodate incurable patients up to one-third of its total patient population, Beauport's proprietors, like Workman, endeavoured on several occasions to admit only recent cases of insanity. They hoped in this way to define their institution as an asylum primarily for the cure of insanity. As we shall see, in both provinces similar explanations would be put forth to rationalize their growing population of chronic patients.

By virtue of their position as proprietors of a monopoly in the state farming-out system, the Beauport directors' outlook on moral treatment and on the issue of curability was ultimately more pragmatic than Workman's. Despite expressing concern about the interrelated issues of the growing chronic-patient population and the tremendous overcrowding at their institution, Douglas, Frémont, and Morrin fought against the establishment of other psychiatric institutions elsewhere in the province. Their blend of entrepreneurial and medical ambition led them to evince less outrage and distress about the disparity between the great promise of moral treatment and the reality of incurability. Although they attempted to incorporate important features of the architecture of moral treatment into their asylum, their agenda was from the outset never entirely compatible with its ideological tenets.

The actual treatment strategies of moral therapy were similar in both Ontario and Quebec. The same combination of patient work, amusement, diet, and daily regimen was seen to be the best means of patient recovery. Superintendents at the Toronto Asylum, like their counterparts at Beauport, believed that the "best course of treatment of the insane [was] that in which the least medicine [was] employed."[47]

Work as therapy was of central importance to the success of moral treatment in both provinces. Work, and the exercise it generated, was recommended both to divert the alienated mind from the morbid associations connected with a patient's insane condition and to regulate the digestive and respiratory systems. In an era in which there was a close diagnostic relationship between a patient's mental and physical condition, work therapy was seen to be of tremendous benefit.[48] The timing and form of the prescribed work was to be subject to the medical expertise of the alienist. As Superintendent Roy of the Beauport Asylum explained: "Work is not suited to all patients, especially to maniacs. It is rarely efficacious at the commencement of the disease and it is even not always suited to [the] ascensional phase of the disease, for it would incur a risk of increasing the agitation. Violent exertion must at all events be altogether avoided, and would occasion more harm than good, and we use it only when the disease has passed its acute stage and threatens to become chronic and result in dementia."[49] Patient work was a repetitive, steady, and orderly activity, that, if properly supervised inside and outside the institution by attendants and medical staff, could re-instill the regular and sober habits that medical superintendents considered essential to patient recovery.

Here the alienists' understanding of the medical benefits of work therapy merged with their social perceptions of rationality and order. As Workman put it, one of the purposes of work therapy was that "many of the patients must leave their places of temporary confinement [as] more useful and independent members of society than they were before becoming insane."[50] Even for chronic patients, whose chances of leaving the asylum were slim, work therapy was seen to provide many rehabilitating benefits. Another rationale for work therapy was that by engaging in work government patients would in varying degrees be earning their keep as privileged inmates of one of society's most benevolent institutions.

In addition to sewing, knitting, and helping with a wide range of domestic activities inside the institution, female patients worked in the laundry, in the kitchen, and as dairy maids on the farm. They helped clean patient rooms and attended to patients less healthy than themselves. Male patients were encouraged to work on the asylum farm and in the garden. They worked at trades such as masonry and carpentry and as manual labourers in the renovations and subsequent additions to the asylums. They also worked in the asylum bakery and the tailor shop, helped engineers to load coal into the asylum furnaces, chopped and transported wood for asylum use, and performed a multitude of other tasks. As asylum infrastructures grew, male patients were also set to work in machine shops.

A less therapeutic and more practical aspect of patient work was the use of patient labour to help offset the costs of asylum maintenance. The extent to which patient work was therapeutic, profitable, or exploitative was subject to debate. The subtle contradictions in the alienists' philosophy of work for both medical and financial considerations were brought to the fore by the occasional dispute between asylum officials and patient families. In 1849, for example, the family of Jean Dupont, a patient in the Beauport Asylum, along with some members of the parish of Beauport, wrote to the provincial secretary insisting that Dupont had for some time recovered his sanity. They argued that, despite his recovery and his expressed desire to go back home to his family and friends, he was being kept in the asylum in a state of "slavery" because he was a good worker whose labour was of great value to the institution. The provincial secretary requested that the asylum commissioners arrange the immediate release of Dupont, adding that he desired no such controversy to arise in the future.[51] For their part, the proprietors of the Beauport Asylum argued that no real profit could be extracted from the labour of patients in the asylum. "The labour of lunatics, generally speaking," they noted, "does not pay."[52]

A similar debate broke out over the work of Henry Jones, a patient who lived at the Toronto Asylum from 1870 until his death in 1907. In February 1894 asylum inspector Christie received an application from Jones's wife, Lucy Jones, "for some compensation for the work [her husband had] done in the tailor shop" during the course of his long stay at the Toronto Asylum. Concerned about the petition, Christie asked the superintendent, Daniel Clark, for a statement as to whether "the patient's employment [had] been constant or if he [was] as efficient as represented" by his wife. Christie ended his letter to Clark by emphasizing that he "had no idea that any compensation [could] be given him, as an acknowledgement in this respect would open up the way to any amount of applications along the same lines."[53]

In his report to Christie, Clark had the following to say about the patient's long work history:

He has been an inmate for 23 years and is a tailor. He has worked in our tailor shop more or less during that period when physically and mentally able to do so. For a number of years he has only worked at intervals as for weeks and months at a time he has not been able to work. His work has been principally at repairing old clothes and in his way he has been useful. He does very little work now and is not likely to do much more as he is getting old and feeble. If the principle of remuneration for such for work is acted upon then there are large numbers here similar to him who would be entitled to consideration.[54]

Writing to the provincial secretary, Christie underlined "the Superintendent's objection to the principle of remuneration to patients for work done in the institutions," arguing that "it would form a precedent that could not be carried out satisfactorily." He further noted that "all patients are encouraged to work in some way for their individual benefit, but the fitful way in which work is performed by them would not warrant compensation." Finally, Christie reassured the provincial secretary about Jones' case: "It does not appear that any extra advantage has been derived from the labour of the patient."[55]

In the face of protests and demands for compensation by relatives, Christie and Clark, like their counterparts in Quebec, de-emphasized the usefulness and value of patients like Jones. Although a patient's insanity could be benefited through work, it was argued, the same mental condition precluded a patient from being considered a legitimate wage earner. It is obvious, however, that in different contexts superintendents and inspectors used patient labour for its considerable potential in reducing the costs of asylum management. Christie strongly encouraged the use of patient labour under the supervision of hired workers in various departments of the Toronto Asylum.[56] Steward John Milligan, in his evaluation of the productivity of the Malden Asylum farm, calculated that the labour of "two patients [was] equal to one able-bodied labourer." On this basis he concluded that "the produce of the farm covers all costs, and gives a very handsome profit also."[57] Asylum attendants were valued by inspectors and superintendents for their ability to maximize the work potential of the patients they supervised. John Kelly, chief tailor at the Toronto Asylum, for example, was praised by Superintendent Clark: "He succeeds well with the patients who work under him." This success resulted in "a great improvement in the amount of work turned out and the quality of work done."[58]

In his report on patient work at the Beauport Asylum, Inspector Wolfred Nelson recommended that, as "several of the females were ... employed [and] as women are naturally given to seek occupation, every effort should be made to provide them with some work as a means of amusement, and to divert their minds from dwelling on imaginary ills." Nelson considered patient work for males and females of importance from both a "remedial and pecuniary point of view."[59] Some superintendents were proud of the amount of food and other supplies that could be produced through supervised patient labour at considerable savings to the institution.[60] It was also common for superintendents to give statistical returns on the productivity of asylum patients at a variety of trades and on the farm.[61] In many cases the quest for profit and the minimization of the costs of asylum maintenance dominated discussions between superintendents and asylum inspectors.[62]

Patient entertainment or amusement was also considered to be integral to the practice of moral therapy in Ontario and Quebec. There were both physical and psychological components to this aspect of patient therapy. Patients, especially those who were unable or who refused to work, were encouraged to take walks around the asylum grounds and play at a number of games, including cricket, croquet, bowling, and billiards, in order to exercise the body. Such exercise was in turn meant to stimulate mental activity.[63] Drama clubs, music clubs, and church choirs were also established, and regularly scheduled dances, lectures, and magic lantern exhibitions were introduced into asylum regimens. Most nineteenth-century asylums in Ontario and Quebec also had libraries with book collections selected to promote "sensible" reading.[64] Beyond the professed therapeutic strategy of patient amusements was the practical need for diversion from the monotony of asylum living. Thus asylum attendants and superintendents themselves were often eager participants in these activities.

The final component to moral treatment was the regular delivery of religious services. At Beauport both Catholic and Protestant services were held. As with work and amusements, religion was seen to have a strong therapeutic component. According to Douglas, Frémont, and Morrin:

Without expressing an opinion concerning the spiritual effects of these religious observances ... we are convinced that they are really important for their curative effects; they can govern the excessive ideas of the mentally ill, settle their restlessness, and inspire in them a distrust of their own illusions. Many patients who are wild and undisciplined in their rooms suddenly become silent and remain attentive and respectful during the service. Old memories, customs, and sensations are rekindled, resulting in a marked improvement.[65]

Religious services had the additional benefit of re-emphasizing customs and practices in which patients had formerly participated while in a sane condition. They also served to instill discipline and order in much the same way as patient work and amusements did.

Historian S.E.D. Shortt has noted that "the treatment protocol of the London Asylum, based on the triumvirate of work, religion, and constructive amusement, was both typical of most Anglo-American institutions and consistent with a pessimistic view of etiology and prognosis," in the late nineteenth century.[66] Although the same tri-partite treatment strategy was practised in the era of the "discovery of the asylum" in Ontario and Quebec, the promise that moral therapy had held out was tempered by actual experiences of patient treatment. As it became increasingly obvious that the high cure rates originally guaranteed by the early proponents of moral therapy would not be achieved in Ontario or Quebec, the proprietors at Beauport and the superintendents at the Toronto Asylum constructed parallel arguments to explain this failing.[67] Without abandoning their faith in the therapeutic potential of moral treatment, they argued that a combination of factors at the pre-committal stage were militating against patient cure in the asylum.

Perhaps the most important explanation among alienists for the increasing numbers of chronic and incurable patients in the asylum in Ontario and Quebec was the timing of patient committal. Subscribing to the prevailing theory of the importance of early treatment, alienists claimed that the longer the delay in getting "lunatics" into the asylum for treatment, the less likely it was that they would recover. Both Workman and the proprietors of the Beauport Asylum asserted that when their institutions first opened they had been forced to accommodate large numbers of patients from local jails and provisional asylums, and that these patients were invariably ones whose mental disorders had been of long standing. According to the principle of early treatment, these patients were unlikely to recover by moral therapeutic means.[68] and the asylums were therefore inhabited by a preponderance of patients with unpromising prognoses.

Further adding to the burden of chronic and incurable patients in asylums were family members sent to the asylum after a prolonged period of care in the home. According to the house physician at Beauport, "in the majority of cases, the families of persons attacked with insanity, swayed by ignorant prejudice, false shame, or weak pity, defer, as long as possible, sending them to the asylum. They thus allow the favourable moment to pass away, when the disease might be easily cured, and the consequence is, that individuals who might have been restored to reason and to society, become the victims of confirmed insanity" in the asylum. Skeptical of the existence or value of any home-based care or therapy, alienists in Ontario and Quebec, as elsewhere, reasoned that prolonged confinement at home denied patients the benefits of early asylum treatment.[69]

If families were to blame for not sending their relations to the asylum early enough for effective moral treatment, local family physicians also frequently came under fire for their unenlightened treatment strategies. According to Workman: "One of the greatest evils connected with the disease is by all medical superintendents of asylums, declared to be the over-treatment of the patients, in the hands of country practitioners. I have had under care a multitude of cases in which indiscreet recourse to blood letting, severe purgatives and other depressive remedies, or the gross abuse of narcotics, has been productive of the most distressing results." Although not casting all local doctors in such an unfavourable light, Workman, like his counterparts in Quebec, was quick to criticize the more traditional medical perceptions and treatments of insanity at the local level for not conforming with the theory and practice of contemporary asylum therapy.[70] Like the families they treated, local practitioners, ignorant of "the approved system of modern therapeutics applicable to its cure," unwittingly consigned many patients to a chronic or incurable state.[71]

A related explanation for low cure rates was the tendency in both provinces for many of the insane to be detained in local district jails before committal to the asylum. After permanent asylums were established in Ontario and Quebec, the removal of the insane from local jails to asylums became a priority, in an effort to relieve the jails of a burden no longer considered appropriate to their function. Because asylums were unable to meet public demand for asylum accommodation, however, local jails remained sites of first committal. As a strategy to get their ailing relatives transferred quickly to the asylum, families would sometimes have them declared "dangerous to be at large" and then confine them in a local jail until a warrant was issued for their transfer to the asylum. The use of this strategy of course offered quick and convenient relief to families. But superintendents for the most part deplored such scheming, arguing that the environment of local jails, and the harsh treatment of patients in them, frequently confirmed rather than improved their mental derangement. The complicated process of committal from the jail to the asylum, they argued, also caused unnecessary legal delays in providing the preferred institutional treatment for the patients.

Alienists also complained that most of the patients who came from local jails, like many who came directly from their community, brought with them insufficient medical information to communicate the nature and extent of their affliction. Although an official medical questionnaire and proper medical certificates were supposed to be sent to the asylum along with the patient being transferred, the necessary information was usually missing. Asylum superintendents claimed that the lack of medical histories limited the efficacy of treatment in the asylum.[72] Workman also charged that, in their haste to have certain people committed, justices of the peace and family members sometimes fabricated medical details that they thought would lead to a faster committal.[73]

Finally, superintendents in both Ontario and Quebec argued that the lack of asylum accommodation for patients also contributed to the ineffectiveness of moral therapy. In both provinces the superintendents reported that the numbers of applicants for admission far exceeded the number that could be accommodated. Although in both provinces measures were eventually taken to restrict admissions to recent cases, superintendents explained that the flood of applicants still necessitated the admission of patients whose disorders had not received expert medical treatment soon enough to prevent aggravation of their condition.

The constellation of interrelated explanations mustered by alienists in both provinces to explain the low cure rates in their respective institutions is important in several respects. Although alientists were forced to acknowledge the low cure rates in their asylums, it is evident that, at least prior to the pessimistic era of degeneration theory, they were not prepared to regard moral treatment as inefficacious therapy. Asylum doctors maintained that moral treatment did effect cures. But they also argued that the possibility of asylum medicine working at its best was thwarted by the social, economic, and cultural realities of the societies in which the respective lunatic asylums were situated.

The societies into which the permanent asylums were born had pre-existing perceptions of, and responses to, insanity. These included various customs of community and family care, treatment by local physicians, and institutional provision in local jails. In their efforts to explain the failure of moral treatment in the asylum, superintendents constructed arguments that essentially blamed the continued use of these more traditional means of treating and managing insanity.[74] The introduction of the lunatic asylum did in some important respects alter the character of earlier perceptions and responses to insanity; but, to the dismay of the medical superintendents, the asylum did not quickly replace them. Asylums tended to become integrated into the network of pre-existing strategies employed to deal with those perceived to be insane.

This process of integration can be illustrated by the case of the district or local jail. Before the introduction of the lunatic asylum, it had been the practice in district jails of Ontario and Quebec to hire a jail physician or surgeon to attend to the medical needs of the inmates.[75] This service included the care of the alleged insane, who were brought to the jail under warrants for petty crimes such as assault or theft, loose, idle, and disorderly conduct, or, most commonly, for being "a dangerous person suspected to be insane."

Despite the introduction of the asylums at mid-century, the local jail continued to be an important institution for the reception of the mentally ill. The commitment of both provinces to rid the jails of their insane inmates ironically guaranteed the perpetuation of the practice of first incarcerating them. An examination of the procedures of the Perth County Jail highlights the local jail's role as a socio-therapeutic setting for the insane well after the introduction of the asylum.[76]

The transfer of a patient from a local jail to the lunatic asylum required several steps. In the case of the Perth Jail, a person suspected of insanity was usually committed to the jail on warrant by one or more justices of the peace. Upon committal the patient was first examined by the jail physician or surgeon, who assessed the patient's physical and mental state and in some cases began a regimen of medical treatment. If the jail surgeon concluded that the patient was insane, he notified the clerk of the peace, who began the process of certification and committal to the asylum. At the Perth County Jail, the clerk of the peace first wrote to the superintendent of the Toronto Lunatic Asylum requesting a copy of the official medical questionnaire that needed to be filled out and sent back to the asylum. This questionnaire, upon which the superintendent would base his subsequent treatment strategy, asked for details related to the medical history of the patient. The completed questionnaire, which contained the medical analysis of the jail surgeon and information gathered from the family or other acquaintances of the patient, was also used to gauge the urgency of the case compared to other requests for committal. The clerk of the peace also alerted three local physicians that their services would be required at the jail for the purposes of evaluating the condition of the patient. If they concurred with the jail surgeon's diagnosis, they filled out a certificate of insanity, a legal document required for committal to the asylum. At this stage, two or more justices of the peace authorized the allocation of funds from the local treasury for transporting the patient from the jail to the asylum. The jail warden or another official was given the responsibility of taking the patient to the asylum along with the pertinent documentation.

This description of the official process of committal from the local jail to the lunatic asylum already hints at the jail's influence on the diagnosis and treatment of insanity. Delays in the committal process could keep patients in the jails for some time, thereby prolonging their treatment by jail surgeons, who, in some cases, developed their own medical outlooks on diagnosis and treatment. Moreover, these procedures make it clear that patients' mental conditions were first determined at the local level. The assessment was based on medical and non-medical information presented by the magistrate(s) who committed the patient, the medical evaluation of the jail surgeon, information derived from acquaintances and relatives who made the decision to commit, and the opinions of the certifying physicians.

The jail surgeon's role could be influential, as reports of the medical treatment of a number of patients by Dr John Hyde, surgeon to the Stratford Jail, illustrate. When Jane Anderson, a Stratford resident, was brought to the jail in a "weak and feeble" state and feeling "low and melancholy," Hyde first administered morphia in order to procure sleep and then instructed the jail attendant to serve her a generous diet. Some time later, he prescribed "cold ablutions thrice daily and quinine and iron" for Anderson's malady.[77] Hyde often combined the treatment of patients' physical disorders with a treatment of their mental disease. Another Stratford Jail inmate, Patricia Peters, was committed by order of the magistrates, "having been found at large." In his first examination of Peters, Hyde noted that she was emaciated and feeble and suffering from chorea, or St Vitus's Dance. The chorea, he observed, subsided in about a week, but was replaced by "excitative madness." For this condition, Hyde administered "five glasses of Portwine daily, and sulphate of morphia to the amount of two grains daily." This prescription enabled Peters to sleep well but did not seem to relieve her insane condition.[78]

In many instances Hyde's treatment appeared successful enough to cure his deranged patients without his having recourse to committal to the Toronto Lunatic Asylum. One such patient, Richard Black, was admitted to the jail in a violent state. According to John Linton, the clerk of the peace, he "could hardly be subdued by the Gaoler and his assistant." Hyde noted that Black was also subject to epileptic fits. Yet during the course of the application procedure for admission to the Toronto Asylum, he reported that Black's condition had improved dramatically and that only in the case of a relapse would he in fact need to be sent to the asylum.[79] Workman did not fail to praise Hyde for his medical efforts, as they occasionally prevented the necessity of a patient's committal to the superintendent's overcrowded asylum. In one instance, Workman expressed his satisfaction that a woman named Davis had recovered under Dr Hyde's care. Her recovery was "another pleasing proof of the fact that judicious treatment might save many patients from the disagreeable alternative of consignment to a Lunatic Asylum."[80] On another occasion, Workman informed the clerk of the peace that one of the jail patients could be sent down to the asylum, "provided [his] good gaol surgeon does not again carry off the prize, a feat in which he has become rather expert."[81]

Although Hyde's therapies often figured prominently in the subsequent fate of a patient first incarcerated in the Perth Jail, the case of John Conrad indicates that the socio-medical world of the local jail encompassed far more than the treatment strategies of its surgeon. Conrad was committed to the jail in February 1858 at the request of his wife. Hyde noticed that Conrad was "really excited" on his arrival and he was informed that the patient had not slept for several nights. Hyde administered "a very large dose of Tincture of Opium in half a tumbler of Port Wine" in hopes of inducing Conrad to sleep thoroughly in the evening. On re-evaluating Conrad's condition the next morning, Hyde found that he had slept well but that his tongue was soft and his pulse "weak and compressible." He ordered that his patient be given a glass of wine four times a day, and a generous diet. After four days of this treatment, Hyde pronounced Conrad cured of his mental alienation and ordered his release from the jail.

After some time at home, however, Conrad was recommitted as insane by the local magistrate. Hyde was informed by Conrad's wife that her husband tended to become very excited "at full moon." Hyde again assessed his patient, this time concluding that he displayed the "well known symptoms of mania à potu," or insanity induced by the overindulgence of "ardent spirits." On the basis of this evaluation, Hyde "resumed the use of wine in connection with sulphate of morphia," which improved Conrad's condition in a few days. Nevertheless, Conrad's wife and some neighbours remained concerned about his mental state and urged his committal to the Toronto Asylum. "Out of a regard to their request," Hyde informed the clerk of the peace, he agreed to add his name to the medical certificate for that purpose.[82] Conrad was subsequently sent to the Toronto Asylum, where he was treated by

Workman for about a month. In correspondence with Linton, Workman mentioned that Conrad's condition had improved to the point where his discharge from the asylum was imminent. Linton responded by strongly urging that Conrad remain in Workman's care for a further period. In Linton's opinion:

I think that your discharging him now, would do away with all the good you have already done him, – as in my non-medical opinion, his nervous system wants a longer "stillness" to make it sounder and stronger to meet the *excitements* of ordinary things in a busy world. You have the means, so far as you can, in your power, and better see him sawing wood, or "chopping stones," or cleaning floors, digging with spades – or anything – *under your care* than his meeting the rebuffs, and uncertainties, and coldness, of a world which *makes* or *creates* nervousness, rather than soothes it – I think, you think so too. I mean, till his nerves are "braver" and a month or so might do that.[83]

On the recommendation of the clerk of the peace, Workman kept Conrad for another month, finally discharging him "at the request of his wife."[84]

Conrad's case indicates that a variety of influences could affect the course of treatment of patients who were taken into district jails. As in many cases the removal of the patient from the context of asylum treatment was ultimately the decision of the family, not the superintendent. A more striking feature of this case was the ability of the clerk of the peace to influence the medical decision of the superintendent on the basis of his own "non-medical" analysis of Conrad's nervous inability to face the excitement of a busy world.

Many cases of purported insanity at the Perth Jail were in fact filtered through the moral universe of the clerk of the peace. Linton frequently gave his opinions and advice to families and acquaintances on the appropriateness of their decision to commit to the jail a person they considered insane. In one instance, John Sparling, a justice of the peace, brought a local woman, Mrs. Steltser, to the jail, noting that she had been for some time "rather outrageous." Sparling expressed concern that Steltser might "do some injury to her family or husband" and asked that she be treated with consideration and offered medical attention in the jail. He strongly recommended her as a fit subject for treatment at the Toronto Asylum, and Linton started proceedings to have her sent to the Toronto

Asylum. But after she had been at the Perth Jail for a few weeks Linton came to quite a different evaluation of her case. Basing his diagnosis in part on the medical report of the jail surgeon, Linton responded to Sparling that:

It is reported to me [by Dr Hyde] that Mrs. Steltser, with kind treatment, would be as well as ordinary people are – and that she is now so. Further, that her husband or any other friend has not come to enquire after her thereby to show some anxiety and humanity for her improvement and recovery. I write this to suggest that it would be better for her husband to see to her state, and to do a husbands duty – and take her home – as it is likely she will be discharged. She is anxious to see her family. There is no vacancy for her admittance in the asylum at Toronto, even if she was a subject for that institution, which I doubt three medical practitioners here would find her to be.[85]

Here, in Linton's view, was a case of spousal and family neglect poorly disguised as a case of insanity. The sheriff of Stratford shared Linton's opinion on this and other cases, noting: "There has been so many patients discharged as cured [by] the Jail Surgeon, [brought] here by the justices for insanity, that I am satisfied such patients should not have been committed at all in the common jail of this county." According to the sheriff, "many justices of the peace throughout the county ... [think] if a complaint is made before them they must commit, right or wrong."[86]

In some instances patients who were diagnosed by the jail surgeon and clerk of the peace as insane and in need of asylum treatment were nevertheless taken back from the jail into the community. Jane Anderson, for example, was committed to the Perth Jail as insane. According to Hyde, she was very reserved and uncommunicative but made a continuous "whining noise," repeating the phrase "Oh! Dear, Oh! Dear." Even though Hyde had recommended her as a fit candidate for the Toronto Asylum, her husband removed her from the jail after five days and took her by railroad to her friends near Whitby in the hopes that "she would thereby get better."[87] Within the same week, another two patients who Hyde thought would have benefited from asylum treatment were retrieved from the jail by relatives.[88]

Through correspondence with the clerk of the peace, acquaintances and relations kept track of the progress of patients in the jail and the asylum. Linton was always prepared to offer his own advice along with any news he had for residents of the district. In one instance, a St Marys resident, John Collins, was committed to the jail as insane by a town constable. A week after his committal, Collins's father sent a letter to Linton requesting the clerk of the peace to "write to [him] once or twice each week" to let him know how his son was "getting about." Linton responded that Collins was "keeping well, ... in his sane mind" and requested that the father send some clean linen to improve the comfort of his son in the jail. Linton added: "If he continues so well, the Dr [Hyde] thinks you may come on Saturday for him."[89] As Collins showed continued signs of improvement, the jail surgeon authorised his discharge shortly thereafter. Upon reaching St Marys, Collins met the constable who had originally incarcerated him. The constable apparently called to Collins, "How did you get out?" Evidently frightened by the constable's challenge, Collins bolted into a nearby wood and disappeared. In a sorrowful letter to the clerk of the peace, Collins's father lamented "the mistake on the part of Dr Hyde in supposing the man to be cured and well in so short a time" and added that he "should of thought the Dr had been more authentically [versed] in the deep planning and scheming to of put my confidence in what these insane men say in their best moods which are commonly of short duration better for me had I of lost the best farm in Canada had I of been the owner of it then he should of been set out at liberty so very soon and alone."[90]

Six months later Collins's father wrote to Linton informing him that his son had resurfaced in the local jail at Sarnia, and asked Linton's advice on how his son could be sent to the Toronto Asylum from the Sarnia Jail. Despite Linton's suggestion that he try to work through the office of the Sarnia Jail in his quest for his son's asylum committal, Collins was back in custody in the Perth District Jail within a month. Soon after Collins's arrival, Linton himself initiated the process of asylum committal. Hyde and two other certifying physicians examined Collins and stated that they "did not consider him then insane" but that: "the tendency to an attack was still existing [as] after his dismissal on the former occasion he indicated dangerous symptoms and [they] decreed it the safer course to grant the necessary certificate in order that he might be placed under the care of Dr Workman for a short period until his recovery would be confirmed which when effected, may prevent a renewal of the attack at least for some time to come."[91]

Shortly after Collins's transfer to the Toronto Asylum, his father again wrote to the district jail inquiring about him. Linton responded that Collins had been transported safely to the asylum by the jail warden, with "special directions sent to the medical superintendent of the Asylum." He added that the jail surgeon had predicted a rapid recovery for Collins under Workman's care and reassuring the father that his "son could not be in a better place to be made well," gave him Workman's address for future correspondence regarding his son's condition.[92]

These examples indicate the role of Ontario district jails in the sometimes complex process of committal both to the jail itself and from the jail to the asylum. As an important medical and social transition point between the community and the asylum, the local jail was an institution through which the needs and perceptions of the community and the medical and moral opinions of jail officials were able to influence the diagnosis and subsequent treatment of insanity. Moreover, the district jail facilitated correspondence between concerned family and acquaintances, and jail detainees and asylum patients.[93]

Local jails in Quebec had similar functions. The physician to the Montreal Jail, Dr Dan Arnoldi, and his successor, Dr Pierre Beaubien, for example, diagnosed and treated as insane many of the jail's inmates. In one case, a young woman whom Beaubien had diagnosed as having an acute form of mania was committed to the jail. Beaubien was particularly concerned that she be sent immediately to the Beauport Asylum as her "affliction" was "strictly one of monomania" and "of recent date." On the basis of his recommendations, the patient was sent to Beauport three days after her arrival at the Montreal Jail. There is evidence to suggest that Beaubien also acted as a correspondent between the Beauport Asylum and the relatives and acquaintances of its patients who had previously been committed to the Montreal Jail.[94] The physicians to the Montreal Jail were responsible for more admissions from jail to asylum than any other Quebec jail physicians. They tended to send several patients to Beauport at once, in a process that involved an appeal to the provincial secretary, who in Quebec had the authority to issue warrants for the transfer of patients to the lunatic asylum.[95]

The physician to the Quebec Jail, from which the second largest number of patients was sent to Beauport, was Dr Joseph Morrin, one of Beauport's proprietors. In his capacity as jail surgeon, Morrin presumably treated and diagnosed cases of madness in ways consistent with his outlook as an alienist.[96] In this capacity Morrin was also able to speed along to the Beauport Asylum cases that he considered to be "recent and curable."[97] But it is evident that some inmates whom Morrin recommended as patients suitable for his asylum were reclaimed by family before they could be transferred.[98]

Some districts in both provinces had no appointed jail physicians to diagnose and treat insanity, but local physicians played a similar role. They would often commit patients to jails in the hopes of manoeuvering a position at the asylum, and they also provided medical attendance at the local jails. As the following example suggests, however, smaller district jails were less experienced in the process of asylum committal. In 1856 a deranged patient, Jean Dubois, was committed to the New Carlisle Jail as dangerously insane. Although there was no hired physician for the New Carlisle Jail, the family physician, Dr. H. Thornton, who had been attending Dubois before his committal to prison, continued to treat him during his incarceration. According to Thornton, Dubois had first manifested symptoms of insanity thirty-five years earlier at the age of fifteen, "on seeing the dead body of a person who fell from a high cliff." The most recent attack of insanity had come as a result of a "fall upon the ice which injured his head" rendering him "insensible for more than half an hour." Although Dubois went through long periods in a "rational and quiet state," these states were interspersed with periods of violence. As Thornton reported, he "destroys his clothes and bedding, reduces himself to a state of nudity, breaks everything within his reach, has a great appetite, sleeps little ... and is dirty in his habits often throwing his excrement at his keepers." In such states, Dubois was put in a straightjacket and handcuffed in order to prevent him from injuring "those who approach him." Thornton appeared to find significant the fact that a sister and a brother of Dubois were also insane, possibly alluding to the idea of hereditary insanity. In the doctor's opinion, "the only chance of his recovery [was] in being sent to an asylum for insane persons."[99]

The sheriff of New Carlisle notified the government of the case but did not enclose any of the official documents needed to initiate Dubois's transfer to the Beauport Asylum. This omission resulted in delays in the committal process that ultimately thwarted the efforts of the sheriff and the family to get appropriate treatment for him. Dubois's health declined "daily" after his incarceration in the local jail and he died there before official consent for his transfer to the asylum was sent from the government to the New Carlisle sheriff.[100]

As the preceding case from the New Carlisle Jail suggests, the threatment methods of the local physician constituted another socio-medical context to be taken into account when studying the perceptions of and responses to insanity in nineteenth-century Ontario and Quebec. Like the local jail, the medical practice of the general practitioner who dealt with cases of insanity was influenced in many ways by the introduction of the lunatic asylum in the provinces. But since local physicians came from a wide range of medical traditions and educational backgrounds, they used a range of medical strategies to deal with insanity, many of which had pre-dated the introduction of the lunatic asylum and its therapeutic ideal.[101] The therapies of the family physician and those of the asylum alienist were therefore not always consistent. Moreover, for a number of reasons, many patients who were being treated in their local communities were not considered to require the medical services of the lunatic asylum. The practices of general practitioners were thus integral to the socio-medical environment for the diagnosis and treatment of insanity of which the asylum became a part after its introduction at mid-century.

On a practical level, the issuing of the medical certificates that were required to commit someone to the lunatic asylum generated considerable business for many local physicians in both provinces. The official cost of a medical examination and certificate of insanity in Ontario was about four dollars. The process of certification by three licensed regular physicians in Ontario or by one or more regular physicians in Quebec, offered in itself a financial incentive for many local doctors to seriously consider the idea of asylum treatment of the insane.

It is also clear that many local physicians believed in the therapeutic promise of the lunatic asylum. In 1867 the family physician to Olivier Bernard, for example, wrote to the government insisting that since it was his patient's "first attack, his illness could perhaps be cured if he were confined to an asylum and underwent treatment, whereas experience has shown that if he remains with his family such a final result cannot be expected."[102] This physician was well versed in alienist arguments about the perils of home care and the need for early asylum treatment. In similar fashion, a local physician from Quebec City urged the quick admission of his patient because: "his illness threatens to become chronic and incurable, whereas if he were placed in an asylum, this young man would have every chance of a rapid and long-lasting cure in the care of asylum staff."[103] In such cases, local physicians clearly believed that the recent or temporary nature of their patients' mental derangement made them promising candidates for asylum therapy.

Some local physicians were noticeably perturbed about their inability, for one reason or another, to send their deranged patients to the asylum for what they considered to be the best treatment. Dr F.L. Gerand of Montreal, while petitioning the government for admission of one of his patients to Beauport, noted that he deeply regretted "the complete lack of any asylum for lunatics in the District of Montreal." In Gerand's view, "simple justice for this part of the country, as well as local needs, requires an establishment similar to the one in Beauport."[104] In another case, Dr Laurendeau, having successfully obtained admission to the asylum for one of his patients, was informed by the patient's parents that they could not bear the thought of their daughter being confined so far away from them. He was furious at the family for refusing to let their daughter be committed: "for the woman was, still is, and probably always will be, deprived of her mental faculties." Laurendeau vowed never to petition again for a patient's committal unless he was certain that both of the patient's parents were "convinced of her madness."[105]

If some local physicians recommended the lunatic asylum for reasons consistent with the therapeutic outlook of its alienist practitioners, others endorsed the asylum for decidedly different reasons. In many cases local practitioners, despite noting the long-standing or incurable nature of their patients' mental illnesses, nevertheless recommended the lunatic asylum as the appropriate medical institution for their treatment. In a petition to have a patient, Alex Johnston, committed to the asylum, for example, Dr M.S. Scott made the following commentary:

I have known him nearly two years, during which time he had been under my care more or less. His disposition when sane is very mild, but when he has his delirious spells, he is often so vicious as to require to be bound. What may have been the cause of his aberration of mind I cannot with any certainty decide – it has been of somewhat long standing and the physicians who treated him in the onset are all dead. He has frequent attacks of epileptic convulsions, after which he generally is insane (after raving) until another epileptic attack which generally leaves him sane. Much of the time however he seems to labor under severe melancholy. On the 19th February last – during one of his melancholy seasons he attempted suicide by cutting his throat – I was by him in a short time and dressed his wounds – he was able to speak and did converse –- but his conversation showed his mind to have been in a sadly perverted state.[106]

Despite the apparent length of Johnston's insanity, his physician recommended him for asylum treatment. Similarly other patients whose insanity was of long standing or who had been labelled "imbecile," "idiotic," or otherwise incurable were nevertheless recommended by their family physicians for asylum treatment, despite asylum policy.[107]

There were several reasons for local physicians' recommending chronic and incurable patients for asylum treatment. In Quebec, this practice stemmed in part from the Beauport Asylum's early policy of taking a certain percentage of incurable cases.[108] Also, much to the chagrin of alienists, local doctors believed that after the failure of their own medical interventions, however lengthy, the asylum was the right institution to manage and treat their patients, regardless of the slim prospects of cure.[109] Finally, community physicians in both provinces tended to combine social and medical rationales in their attempts to get patients sent to the asylum. Integral to the socio-medical role of family doctors was a familiarity with the social and economic circumstances in which their patients lived. Local physicians therefore often regarded the asylum as both a medical facility and a social institution for the relief of a range of socio-medical ills.

In his effort to have one of his patients committed to the asylum, Dr John Fitzpatrick from Quebec City noted that the man in question was "quite idiotic and incapable of taking care of himself." Fitzpatrick further noted that his patient was "in a state of extreme poverty and ... chiefly supported by the society of St Vincent de Paul."[110] In a similar Quebec petition, Dr Wolfred Nelson wrote to the government about a patient in need of asylum care: He "has been in a state of idiocy for the last seventeen years. He is an orphan ... and for many years has been taken care of by his uncle ... who being in very declining circumstances is totally unable to maintain him any longer."[111] In another case, a patient who had experienced the beginnings of paralysis ("great weakness in his lower extremities and pain and fatique the length of his spinal cord") was sent to the Hôtel Dieu in Montreal after unsuccessful treatment by his local doctor, Dr Paquin. According to Paquin, the over-administration of strychnine in his patient's treatment at the hospital had only aggravated his mental illness and within a short period of his discharge from hospital to his home, he was completely insane and had lost the use of his legs. Paquin requested his patient's quick transfer to the asylum in order to prevent his wife from succumbing to the fatigue that resulted from providing and caring for her husband and their seven children.[112] As these and other examples indicate, the rationales of local physicians' for the need for asylum committal could be as social as they were medical.

On the other hand, many patients diagnosed as insane were not necessarily considered by their family physicians to be candidates for the therapy of the lunatic asylum. Historian Jacalyn Duffin notes that Dr John Langstaff, during his forty years of medical practice in Ontario, treated twenty-nine patients whom he diagnosed as having severe mental illness, fifteen who were less severely afflicted, eight who had attempted or committed suicide, and about fifty "who suffered predominantly psychiatric symptoms as part of another physical disorder."[113] Of these, Langstaff certified only nine as suitable candidates for the lunatic asylum. The rest he treated in his home visits according to the therapeutic regimen of his "orthodox" medical outlook. Langstaff's treatment of his mentally ill patients suggests that he considered them to exhibit a broad range of deranged mental states. His medical strategies, including the use of sedatives, laxatives, electrostimulation, and comforting repeat visits, reflected the complex variety of symptoms he observed and his own medical outlook as a mid-nineteenth-century physician.[114]

Langstaff's treatment of patients who he considered to be suffering from mental alienation illustrates the diversity of socio-medical responses to insanity in Ontario and Quebec. The nineteenth-century medical practitioner tended to a large number of patients who were considered to be mentally deranged. Nevertheless, only a fraction of those patients underwent the systematic moral treatment of the lunatic asylum. Asylum superintendents would most likely have been highly critical of Langstaff's disinclination to recommend many of his patients to the asylum. Furthermore, as evidence from other local physicians suggests, when country practitioners did decide to commit, it was often for reasons inconsistent with the medical principles of asylum treatment.

The diagnoses and treatment regimens of Langstaff and other physicians were part of a range of socio-therapeutic approaches in Ontario and Quebec that was influenced by, and interrelated with, the rise of the lunatic asylum. However, many of their approaches were incompatible with the alienist social and medical outlook. Ironically, the persistence of these non-asylum contexts formed the basis of the alienists' explanations for the failure of the therapeutic promise of the asylum in both provinces.

Further militating against the realization of the superintendents' vision of the asylum as the proper therapeutic environment for the treatment and cure of insanity as a medical disorder were the social, economic, and political contexts of committal. The following examination of the decision to commit at the lay, or community level, indicates the extent to which the asylum was not in essence a medical institution as traditionally defined. The circumstances precipitating committal were often antithetical to the philosophy of the asylum as an institution for the moral regulation and medical treatment of insanity. In many respects, the relatives and neighbours of those considered insane took advantage of the lunatic asylum in ways not originally intended by alienists and asylum advocates. Nevertheless, this discrepancy did not preclude a direct relationship between those who wanted to arrange a committal and those who held power and authority in government and asylum administration. Individual decisions at the local level were inextricably linked to the decisions of state and asylum officials.

4 Wanderer, Pauper, and Prisoner: The Social, Economic, and Political Contexts of Committal

Towards the end of July, 1852 James Hardey, a farmer at Niagara Falls, was approached by a young woman he had never before seen. Hardey described her as "most pitiable ... being weakened by dysentery and loathsome with vermin." Her behaviour was "sometimes quiet, and sometimes quite outrageous." Not having the heart to drive the stranger off "in such a state," Hardey took her in and kept her for five weeks while he tried to locate her family. After the woman told him that her father ran a tavern in Dunville, Hardey wrote to her father informing him of his daughter's whereabouts, but he received no reply. A few days later, the stranger told Hardey that she thought her father made baskets but she didn't know where.

Having no luck locating the woman's family, Hardey next wrote to the Niagara Falls Municipal Council requesting that they send her to the lunatic asylum in Toronto. The councillors replied that the asylum had been recently "shut against those who [were] unable to pay their way through it and [that the council had] ... no funds at their disposal for any such purpose."[1] This rejection prompted Hardey to write a letter to the government protesting how unreasonable it was that he should have to pay taxes towards an institution that did not admit pauper patients. He insisted on an order for the admission of the stranger to the Toronto Asylum where, through proper treatment, she might be "restored to her right mind." The provincial secretary responded that while the power of accepting applications was vested solely in the Board of Commissioners, the asylum's prohibition against pauper patients had since been withdrawn. Upon receiving this news, Hardey sent the woman off to Toronto with neighbouring farmers, Mr and Mrs Imlay, in the hopes of securing the woman's committal to the asylum there.[2]

When they arrived in Toronto, the Imlays called at the residence of asylum commissioner Reverend John Roaf. As he had just returned to Toronto from a trip to England, Roaf could not tell the Imlays whether the ban on government patients had been lifted. He was therefore hesitant to sign an order for the woman's admission to the asylum and suggested that the Imlays raise the matter with commissioner William McMaster at his residence. McMaster in turn informed the Imlays that he was under the impression that the asylum was still closed to pauper patients. He referred them to Dr Christopher Widmer, the chairman of the Board of Commissioners, but added that it was unlikely that Widmer would sign the woman over to the asylum since he had "used his influence to have the Asylum shut against those for whose benefit it was principally intended." Having no luck with Dr Widmer, the Imlays proceeded to the asylum itself to convince the superintendent to commit their charge. There they were simply informed that the price of admission was six pounds and six shillings for a quarter of a year's "maintenance." The Imlays again tried Commissioners Roaf and McMaster but were unable to contact them at their residences.

Finally they proceeded to the residence of yet another commissioner, Mr [John] Patterson. Reporting on their conversation, Mr Imlay concluded: "I should have been mistaken if I had left the city with the idea that the chairman and all the members of the Board of Directors were alike insane, for [Patterson] kindly consented to sign the document required for the admission of the Patient, on condition that I would promise, when I went to the asylum, to pay ten shillings for her week's maintenance and give my note for the remaining six pounds." Patterson reassured Imlay that he would never be asked to pay the six pounds and that the note was just a formality to initiate the admission proceedings. Thus, after two weeks of begging, the Imlays were finally able to commit the female stranger to the asylum on the evening of 11 October 1852.[3]

This example of the long route to asylum committal, although specific in some respects, is representative of the complex social, economic, and political forces that came to bear on the decisions of family, friends, and neighbours to commit others to the lunatic asylums of Ontario and Quebec. While the asylum may have been originally conceived and subsequently administered by reformers and alienists with a particular socio-medical agenda in mind, it soon became an institution that responded also to a wide range of lay needs at the local level of Canadian society in the nineteenth century.

The complex process of family- and community-initiated asylum confinement has been the focus of several recent studies.[4] Considering the findings of all these studies, historian David Wright has argued that the driving force behind asylum development in the nineteenth century was the decision to commit made by the family.[5] He suggests that the changes in the family brought on by industrialization influenced motivations for committal and were central to asylum development. Moreover, in Wright's view, the "non-educated masses [were unlikely to] cast off centuries-old cultural and popular ideas about insanity when confronted by the medical gaze" of the superintendent and his asylum. The findings of my analysis of the motivations for committal of pauper patients to the asylum follow from those of Wright's analysis in two fundamental respects. First, in Ontario and Quebec there is little evidence to suggest that during the nineteenth century decisions to commit made at the local level ever became medicalized according to the logic of asylum alienists. Second, demand for asylum accommodation was predominantly fuelled by requests for committal at the local level, either by individual families or by community representatives.

However, as influential as decisions at the local level were in shaping the process of asylum development, they cannot be studied in isolation from the decisions of those who wielded authority at the asylum and state levels in the provinces. Asylum accommodation may have been locally driven, and the asylum may have become "the arbiter of social and familial conflict."[6] But even if the process of committal was initiated at the local level, it could not be enacted without the involvement of the complex power structures of the state and the fledgling alienist profession in asylum development. Family and community motivations for committal must therefore be considered in the wider context of alienist and state interests.

One of the greatest pressures precipitating the decision to initiate committal procedures in Ontario and Quebec was socio-economic hardship. In both provinces, one of the prerequisites for admitting a pauper patient to the asylum was the inability of the patient or the patient's family and friends to contribute towards the costs of institutional maintenance. It was inevitable that proof of such penury would be required in the petition for committal. In fact the state was quick to contest the financial distress of families that it considered able to afford to participate in the expenses of asylum care. In one example, the provincial secretary stated flatly to a local justice of the peace: "It would appear that the family of Mr. McDonald is far from being in a destitute condition and is able to contribute if not for the whole at least for a certain share of the expense attending to his support in the above mentioned establishment. You will therefore be so good as to acquaint me to what amount Mr McDonald's family is able to contribute towards his maintenance in the asylum – the pay thereof to the government to be secured by a bond to His Majesty before his admission."[7] In many instances, however, it was clear that the crushing pressure of poverty and not merely the inability to pay for asylum care led to the decision to commit individuals as pauper patients.

Frequently the prolonged mental instability of the principal wage earner of a family led to a petition for committal. In one case, the five-year bout of insanity of a journeyman from St Jacques de l'Achigan led to prolonged poverty for his large family, which had "been reduced to the direst straits and was dependent on local charity for its subsistence." The journeyman's wife, continually hoping that he might recover his sanity, had tried to care for him at home. But with his steady deterioration and the increasing desperation of the family's poverty, she finally petitioned for her husband's committal to the Beauport Asylum.[8] In a similar case, James Dooley from Sorel, the principal male wage earner of a large family already "in indigent circumstances," became insane, leaving his family "in a state of utter misery." The local priest sent him to the Montreal General Hospital, but Dooley returned a month later recovered in body but "more disordered than ever" in mind. With the mother of the family "on the eve of confinement, and the family destitute of the commonest necessities of life," Dooley was committed to the lunatic asylum.[9]

With the onset of mental alienation, the breadwinner's inability to provide for a family increased the burden of work for the spouse and other family members. Jane Carlisle of Montreal, for example, in a petition to the government, explained that her husband had for some time "been diseased in mind, and in consequence [was] unable to provide for the wants of [herself] and her family," which consisted of five children. Carlisle had increased her workload as a washerwoman in an effort to make up for the loss of her husband's income. But the "labour consequent upon her occupation and the care and constant attention demanded by her husband," in addition to the care of her children, were "wearing in the extreme," finally prompting her to ask for her husband's admission to the lunatic asylum. Carlisle assured the government that such an act of "clemency" would "enable her to procure for herself and her children the means of support by her own exertions."[10]

The "gender of breadwinners"[11] of course varied from family to family. Three seamstresses from Quebec "struggled for many years ... to support an aged mother [who was] infirm and blind." As the sisters grew older, "their means of maintenance ... diminished as the demands of filial duty increased," until the youngest and best seamstress of the family became "afflicted with mental derangement of an aggravated kind." The consequent loss of revenue and the additional burden of care that fell to the other sisters led them to initiate proceedings for their deranged sister's committal to the asylum.[12]

The family disruption resulting from the mental affliction of the female head of a household could also lead to a decision to commit. A farmer, Abraham Deignault, noted in his petition for committal of his wife that for a period of four or five years she had been "deranged in mind," and that in the constant struggle to maintain her family of five children her affliction had worsened to the point where she was a terrible burden on the family. In her degenerated state, she had set fire to their barn, destroying a large quantity of hay and grain along with a horse, carts, and harnesses. Exasperated, Deignault appealed to the government, stating: "The continued watchfulness required to prevent evil has impeded your petitioner in the necessary cultivation of his farm upon which the maintenance of his family solely depends[,] and now being destitute of this year's crop as well as under the necessity of begging to assist him in rebuilding his barn stables and likewise to beg for the support of his children he is driven to the necessity of applying that his unfortunate wife should be admitted to the asylum."[13] Similarly, a journeyman, H. Roy, was only able to earn a portion of his wages as he was "obliged to spend a fair amount of his time at home as a result of his wife's madness." "Home" in his case was the immigrant sheds of Faubourg, Quebec. This family's increasing economic hardship led to some of their children being sent to an orphanage in Montreal to prevent them from dying of hunger.[14] In both cases it was the devastating impact of the insanity of the female head of the family that prompted recourse to the asylum.

The downward spiral of economic fortune that eventually precipitated committal to the asylum often resulted from families exhausting their financial means on home and local care. Niagara resident William Noel, for example, noted that his "pecuniary resources [were] entirely inadequate in consequence of the situation of his son, and even the limited means he had [were] very much reduced by the expenses incidental to the endeavours he [had] made to effect the cure of his son" at home. Noel assured the provincial secretary that "it was not till every means within his reach had failed to effect his son's relief that he could consent to present his [son's] case before" the government.[15] Similarly, George Johnston of Valcartier, Quebec applied for the committal of his wife, having run out of funds with which "to employ persons to mind her in his absence."[16]

While some families resorted to the lunatic asylum only after the expenses of home care became overwhelming, others requested asylum relief because of the immediate circumstances of their dire poverty.[117] This was especially the case when the caregivers of the insane were themselves supported by public charity. In one case, the community members of St Catherine in Quebec were of the opinion that a father and his son were both insane. But while the father was sociable and clean enough in his personal habits to be kept under the continued care of neighbours, his son was "so intolerable that no one would go out of their way to take him in."[18] The neighbours therefore asked for his committal to the asylum. In other instances, a single mother, father, sister, or brother who already relied on public charity for support found it impossible to care for a relative who had become deranged.[19] In such desperate cases, it was argued, "in the asylum they would at least be given bed, board, and clothing and would not fear, as they do now, dying of cold or starving."[20]

Other stresses in the family or the community often combined with economic pressures to determine a decision to commit. In many communities, orphans who were perceived to have lost their reason posed particularly difficult problems. In most instances orphans already received some form of local charitable relief. The asylum seemed to many to be a ready-made solution for an orphan who had become mentally deranged. As the Bishop of Quebec described the circumstances of Helen Croft, for example: She "has been for many years an orphan – and has lived with a number of different families in service – for a great length of time in my own – but her growing eccentricities proceeding from aberration of mind have latterly produced a necessity for her continually changing her place, and have fully assumed the character which ... make it imperative to place her under restraint."[21] Thus the bishop advised Croft's admission to the Beauport Asylum. Another orphan, who had been raised by a neighbour, had a sudden onset of insanity that, according to the local parish priest, made it impossible for the neighbour to continue caring for her. Other orphans, boarded out to families by the local community, could be considered unmanageable burdens when suffering from "idiocy" or "mental derangement."[22] Some orphans, among others who were considered insane, found themselves incarcerated in local provincial jails where efforts were made to have them transferred to the lunatic asylum.[23]

Many made the decision to commit because they felt too old and worn out to carry on in their care of those who they perceived as "idiotic" or "insane." In a typical and particularly touching case, Philipe Proux asked for the committal of his thirty-eight-year-old daughter and his thirty-year-old son, noting: "I have supported these children for a great many years, never wishing to commit them to the Beauport Asylum or to ask for a place for them no matter how poor I might be. But now I am poor and old; and, my wife who I counted on to watch these children with care is now ill, aged, and unable to perform this difficult task. I am therefore obliged to beg you to find a place for my two children at Beauport Asylum as government patients."[24]

Louis Magé, another petitioner, had for fifty years cared for a stranger to the community in which he lived, who was considered to be insane. Although Magé had given the stranger "all the care he needed, to the extent that [his] health and circumstances permitted," he informed the government that he was now old and unable to tend to his voluntary charge. Magé added that, as his patient was himself old and epileptic, he probably would not last long as a government patient in the asylum.[25] Jane Wood, a widow, informed the government that she was "worn out with fatigue and distress" from looking after her family of five children, one of whom had been "deranged in mind" for two years. In an effort to relieve her situation, she petitioned for her son's committal to the asylum.[26]

The advanced age or fatigue of caregivers faced with the uncontrollable behaviour of a person considered insane could prompt an appeal for committal. In one such case, Louis Massé and his wife had for many years been looking after their son whom they perceived to be insane. But during a two-month period his insanity became more acute. He was convicted of a minor assault on a neighbour and imprisoned for a short time in the local jail. Upon his release, he continued "to behave in the same dangerous and criminal way as he had previously done, to the point that it became necessary to restrain him, which made him furious." Considering themselves too old to continue managing their son in such a state, his parents saw no option but to appeal for his admission to the asylum.[27]

Increasingly unmanageable behaviour frequently triggered a decision to commit. Father Mignault, from Chambly, Quebec, asserted that a member of his parish who had been periodically insane during the previous fifteen years, had become "more and more dangerous and disturbing for society." Concerned for the safety of his parishioners, Mignault recommended his committal to the asylum.[28] The violent or threatening behaviour of those considered insane was controlled by several methods of confinement. Petitioner Pierre Laurent, for example, in his request for an asylum bed for his son, described his son as mad and dangerous to the point that he had been forced to chain his son's feet to subdue him.[29] Inappropriate behaviour was also a decisive factor. The propensity of some to take off their clothes, to appear in a constant state of filth, or to display other forms of behaviour considered embarrassing or unacceptable could lead to a request for their committal.[30]

Communities often considered the asylum as an expedient refuge for women whose mental breakdown was linked to desertion, as the case of Agathe Valière illustrates. After living for several years in the United States, Valière moved with her husband and children to a small village outside of Montreal. Her husband began suddenly to absent himself from the village for long periods of time, leaving her to rely on public charity to provide for her family. According to reports, this treatment took a severe toll on Valière's sanity. Finally, on a return trip to the village, her husband sold his house and furniture, and absconded to the United States in the middle of the night with his children abandoning "his poor deranged wife in a highly demented state." Allowing Valière to remain in the empty house sold by her husband, the community took turns bringing her food. But eventually her condition deteriorated to the point that they decided to petition the government for her committal to the asylum.[31]

The fragmentary nature of information available in such desertion cases makes the stories of the women in question difficult to piece together. Another story of abandonment leading ultimately to committal emerged from the community of St Michel d'Yamaska. In May 1851 a resident noticed a woman who appeared stranded on the deserted island of St Jean in the Yamaska River. A local navigator took a boat out to the island and found the woman in a state of starvation. He brought her back to shore, but on disembarking, she ran away, jumped into a nearby lake, and swam out some distance. Again the navigator retrieved her, this time placing her under the care of Olivier Stream, one of the community residents. The beleaguered woman told Stream's wife that she had been abandoned by her husband, who now lived in Barnston with another woman. She had been pregnant when found and gave birth while in the care of the residents of Yamaska; but the child died shortly afterwards. Stream noted that although the woman was "absolutely inoffensive" except for her habit of constantly smoking her pipe she was nevertheless decidedly insane. Her madness was allegedly manifested by her preference for her own ragged garments over the new clothes and shoes community members offered her, and by her constant habit of disappearing from her residence at night to wander the nearby roads in all kinds of weather. Although the woman stayed with the Streams for a year and a half, they became uncomfortable with her increasingly eccentric behaviour and by the thought that she might perish if her wandering continued during the coming winter. In November 1852 they petitioned the government for her committal to the asylum.[32]

Many men and women who had been deserted in one way or another became "wandering fools" in the communities of Quebec and Ontario. Indeed, deranged wanderers were still very much a part of the rural landscape in both provinces in the mid-nineteenth century. After asylums were introduced, their communities sometimes tried to have them institutionalized. By taking such action, communities demonstrated varying degrees of benevolence and harsh expedience. Elizabeth Brown was considered by many of the inhabitants of Hemmingford to be insane, wandering and sleeping on the neighbourhood roads. But she was sometimes taken in by residents and offered food and a night's sleep. According to the local parish minister, Gerald O'Grady, however, over time her behaviour had become increasingly unacceptable: she had "broken several windows and ... become a great nuisance." O'Grady felt that her committal to the asylum would be "a great charity to herself and a blessing to the country at large."[33]

In another case, the community expressed considerably less tolerance for a homeless man who wandered from parish to parish begging for his subsistence. He lived for a time in an abandoned cabin where once, in an epileptic fit, he fell onto the stove and badly burned his face and hands. When he wandered from his cabin to a nearby parish to beg, some community members burned down his shelter to deter him from returning to their neighbourhood. According to Father Charles Tardif, parish priest, residents were afraid of his violent and insane behaviour and were worried about the negative impact that his presence might have on the unborn children of pregnant women who saw him in his fits of insanity. Shortly before sending a petition for the stranger's committal on behalf of his parish, Tardif noted with alarm that his worst fears had been realized by the manifestation of an identical form of insanity in a child born of a local woman who had been frightened by the wanderer during one of his epileptic fits. For the community, the asylum was the most expedient means to rid itself of his continued presence.[34]

Some wanderers had family close at hand who either refused to provide the necessary care or felt incapable of providing it. John McGillivray, a justice of the peace from Glengarry, was frequently asked by local residents to take action to prevent "a poor unfortunate man bereaved of his mental faculties" from "roaming about at large." McGillivray was reluctant to confine the wanderer to the local jail, feeling this to be a "very unfit place for a person of his reason." He tried to persuade the parents of the insane man to take action to commit him to the Toronto Temporary Lunatic Asylum. On inquiring into the matter, however, the parents were told that the long duration of their son's insanity prevented him from being admitted to that institution. In response to intensified complaints from the community that the wanderer was getting "more malignant, and mischievous in disposition," McGillivray made a formal petition to the government for his committal.[35] Another such case involved François Jules of Terrebonne. Jules was often found wandering the streets naked or frightening those around him during fits of insanity. Because his father was too poor to keep him confined indoors and give him the attention that his insane condition warranted, the residents petitioned the government to find a place for him in the asylum.[36]

Allusion to the powerful archetype of the wandering fool could in itself form the central argument in a petition for committal. Describing a man who was formerly a respectable clerk and assistant to some of the storekeepers of Armstown but who was said to have recently become insane, local minister W. Brethour warned: Unless the clerk "obtains admission into the [asylum], he will become a wanderer in the country and a terror to anyone to whom he approaches."[37]

The experience of many wanderers highlights the way the community, local jail, and lunatic asylum functioned as a network in the management and social control of insanity in the nineteenth century. In 1843 George Hughes's son, John, fell ill with a condition that developed into insanity over two years. Hughes paid for the services of four different "medical gentlemen" in an effort to cure his son, but this strategy proved both ineffective and expensive. In 1845 Hughes committed John to the Toronto Temporary Lunatic Asylum, but the son was discharged a year later as incurable. Finding his son's violent and destructive behaviour intolerable, Hughes applied to a local justice of the peace for an order for John's "safe keeping" in the local jail near Lancaster. From there, John was sent on to the Toronto Asylum. In May 1847, however, he escaped to New York State where he "roamed about ... till he crossed the river and came back to" his father's residence. Hughes looked after him for a few

days but soon had him recommitted to the local jail while he petitioned for John's readmission to the asylum. Three weeks later,
John once more became a patient at the Toronto Asylum.[38] In this
and other cases, the local prison and the lunatic asylum served as
important institutional components of a loosely integrated system
of care and control when home care or the services of the local
physician were found to be ineffective.

Severe poverty or financial distress, as well as the embarrassing or
disruptive behaviour of those considered to be insane, were the
interrelated circumstances which most often prompted the decision
to commit pauper patients to the state lunatic asylums of Ontario
and Quebec. After the decision to commit was made, however,
there often remained considerable uncertainty about the virtues of
the lunatic asylum itself. This uncertainty resulted in a wide range
of responses on the part of family and community to the state's
acceptance of a petition for asylum committal. In many cases the
offer of asylum accommodation was turned down by the family or
community. Because the demand for asylum accommodation in
Ontario and Quebec far exceeded institutional capacity, there was
often a long delay between the original petition for committal and
its approval by the state. In the interim, the circumstances that had
led to the decision to commit could have considerably changed.

In some cases, by the time approval was granted, the condition of
the intended asylum patient was seen by the family and community to have improved to the point that they no longer saw a need for
asylum treatment or management. In July 1851 for example, Denis
Stevenson petitioned for the committal of his father who had "for
several years been lunatic, and since five weeks [had] been so dangerous that [he was] obliged to keep him chained down in the house
to prevent his doing mischief." After a wait of eleven months the
provincial secretary informed Stevenson that "the next vacancy" at
the Beauport Asylum would be reserved for his father. But Stevenson responded that his father had "taken a sudden turn for the better of late" and that he would therefore "rather have him at home
than at the asylum."[39]

A similar case involving quite different circumstances concerned
a man who left his family to work on the shanties in Ottawa. His
employment had been cut short by a "severe" axe wound that
forced him to return home. Shortly after his return, "symptoms of

insanity began to betray themselves" and, according to his parents, "he became so alarmingly violent and dangerous that it became necessary to have him secured and hourly watched" by volunteers in the neighbourhood. His family and (possibly the community), eventually resorted to sending him to the Montreal Jail "for safe keeping." While in jail he became calmer, but his parents were anxious to have him transferred to the asylum where they hoped that "under proper treatment in a short time his malady might be wholly subdued." Six months after they had petitioned, they were informed that there was a vacancy in the asylum. But they then notified the provincial secretary that their son had "since recovered" and they thus declined the government's offer.[40]

Practical difficulties of transportation from outlying areas to Toronto and Quebec during the winter also led to second thoughts about asylum petitions. The closing of navigation during freeze-up, or a concern about exposing relatives to the perils of winter weather induced many families whose petitions had been accepted to reject offers of committal.[41] If the acceptance was issued before the spring breakup, the government sometimes agreed to reserve the space until the weather permitted the patient's transportation to the asylum. Despite this leniency, however, some families still changed their minds. While grateful for the approval of their petition to have their son committed to the asylum in the late winter of 1853, the Taffards from Montreal, for example, decided to wait: "It will be out of their power to profit by your goodness [the provincial secretary] if the vacancy is not preserved for them until the opening of the navigation as it would be impossible for them to convey their son so long a journey by land in consequence of their poverty and the ungovernable character of the insane man who at times is quite violent and outrageous."[42] Under these circumstances, the government consented to reserve a position, but by the summer of the same year, it was informed that the Taffards had lately "come to the resolution of keeping their son under their own power."[43] Although no acknowledgement of the improvement of their son is apparent in this case, the Taffards nevertheless had second thoughts about their earlier decision to commit.

Conflict between various community members or between community representatives and the family could also lead to the reversal of an earlier decision to commit. Dr J.D. Laurendeau of St Cuthbert petitioned the government for the committal of Ulise

Vallière, who, in the opinion of her husband and her physician, had
become insane. The petition was quickly granted. But two months
later the patient had still not been sent to the asylum. In a letter to
the provincial secretary, an embarrassed Laurendeau explained that
he had learned that Vallière's parents "were keeping her in St. Cuthbert, and wouldn't consent to her being so far away from them."
Vallière's parents did not agree with the doctor or their son-in- law
and preferred to keep their daughter under their own care at home.
This greatly angered Laurendeau, who had gone to great lengths to
have the woman committed to the asylum and remained convinced
of his diagnosis.[44]

Reverend W. King petitioned for the committal of "a young
woman of unsound mind" whom he had encountered on his circuit
duties in St Margaret. Again, the petition was quickly granted, but no
admission followed for several months. When asked about the situation, King informed the government that he was having great difficulty contacting the "poor brother and sister who [had] charge" of
the insane woman. Although her caregivers appeared to be interested in taking advantage of the asylum position offered their sister, they
seemed somehow incapable of being decisive in the matter. After two
warnings from the provincial secrtary that the allocated space would
be given to someone else unless immediate action was taken, communication between King and the government ceased.[45]

Uncertainty about committal could surface even after a relative
had been sent off to the asylum. For a variety of reasons, some
insane individuals were taken out of asylums by family members
and acquaintances well before medical superintendents pronounced
them cured.[46] By law, in both provinces the insane could be discharged into the care of family and acquaintances as long as the
asylum alienists did not consider their being at lasrge to be dangerous to the public. As the demand for admissions was constantly
pressing, they sanctioned most petitions for removal. In some
instances, patients' families considered them sufficiently recovered
to warrant removal after just a short asylum stay. In a petition for
the removal of Jacques Fortin from the St Jean Lunatic Asylum, for
instance, Fortin's family expressed its confidence that his condition
was much improved and that his return home would rehabilitate
him completely.[47] Such family confidence in the rehabilitation of
their relatives could, however, be short-lived, as another case illustrates. Under the impression that his brother had "recovered his

mind" after his six-month stay at the Beauport Asylum, Jean Martin had him released. But a short time later, he petitioned for his brother's recommittal, because he had fallen into the same insane state.[48] Several patients who were officially released as "cured" by asylum superintendents were also sent back to the asylum when the social, economic, and medical circumstances leading to their committal resurfaced.[49]

The uncertainty and strife that could accompany the confinement of family members in a nineteenth-century lunatic asylum are plainly evident in the case of the daughter of a circuit minister in St Sylvestre. In November 1855 Charles Duncan petitioned for the committal of his eldest daughter, Gail, whose mind had by "divine intervention" been "greatly injured." Constantly on the road performing religious services in neighbouring communities, Duncan was unable to help his wife care for his deranged daughter and his "household of ten persons." Duncan's petition was quickly granted by the state. But, within a month of Gail Duncan's arrival at the asylum, the young woman expressed to her mother her "ardent desire to return home." Upon visiting her daughter, Mrs Duncan was distressed by her "wasted frame" and decided to remove her from the asylum. Yet only a few days later, Charles Duncan petitioned for his daughter's recommittal, and this second petition was also accepted. During Gail's eight-month stay at the asylum, her mother visited her and again decided that her daughter would be better off at home. Her second removal from the asylum was partly based on the advice of the asylum warden, Mr Wakeham, who expressed his opinion that "from the strong desire that Miss Duncan manifested to return to the parsonage [such a move] might be the means of her mind regaining its wonted powers, as he had known it in many cases to produce this desirable object." The daughter remained at home for about twelve months, but, in a now familiar pattern, Charles Duncan eventually petitioned to the provincial secretary: "Being frequently from home for a fortnight at a time as a missionary [has made it] next to impossible to manage her any longer at home: the smallness of the house: the sad effect it has had upon her mother's health and spirits and that of the children's make it an imperative duty that I should notwithstanding my many objections yield to the entreaties of all the members of the family and again to send her away." Duncan's petition was quickly approved, and his daughter once again became an asylum patient.[50]

As the Duncan family case suggests, uneasiness about the welfare of a patient in the asylum could motivate the request for removal. Such uneasiness was also evident in the husband of Sophie Mercier, who worried that his wife was not interested in eating or drinking in the asylum. He petitioned through a local priest to take her back, noting his intention to construct a separate room within his house for times when she needed to be confined.[51] One patient, who had been sent from the Montreal Jail to the St Jean Asylum as a "dangerous and violent lunatic" in 1866, had, according to asylum superintendent Howard, become "quiet and tranquil" under his care but was also in an extremely bad state of physical health. The patient's family requested his removal from the asylum so that he could die in the comfort of his home environment. Howard and the provincial secretary saw no objection to the request.[52]

The continued concern that many families expressed over the welfare of those they committed to the asylum, was of course not universal. A large number of patients who were committed formed part of the critical mass of asylum inmates – never visited and never removed – that the superintendents referred to as incurable. They were left to be managed within the newly formed state institutions until they died.

An examination of motivations for committal at the local level reveals that patients were sent to the asylum for reasons grounded more in the social and economic realities of the community and the family than in the socio-medical logic of alienist philosophy. As some historians have pointed out, this discrepancy in turn suggests that some families and communities used the asylum for their own purposes, in accordance with their respective perceptions – social, economic, or medical – of mental derangement. But decisions at the local level were seldom free from the influence of those in power in government or the upper echelons of asylum administration. The great majority of those who petitioned the government for committal had played no part in the reform process that led to the establishment of asylums, or in the articulation of the principles governing asylum development. The decisions of the community (and the fate of the insane) were subject to the influence and interference of asylum and state officials in a number of ways.

At a basic level petitions for committal to the asylum could be severely affected by changes in state policy. In both provinces, during periods in which asylums were greatly overcrowded, delays from three weeks to three years could occur between a petition for committal and its approval by the government. Long waiting periods could greatly increase the hardship of families and communities whose decision to commit had been motivated by extreme economic or social stress. During times when asylum beds were scarce, the administration demanded detailed applications with all necessary documentation before even considering a request for committal. When asylum accommodation was more readily available, however, applications were rapidly accepted. In such periods (for example, after the opening of a renovated portion of the Beauport Asylum), government officials in Quebec commonly granted incomplete petitions, asking only that the appropriate medical documentation be forwarded with the patient to the asylum. During these brief periods, families and community members did not have to work to convince the state of the legitimacy of their cases. The sporadic nature of asylum growth had a significant impact on the local context of committal.

More devastating still to many families was the decision in both provinces, in different periods, to refuse to admit "incurable" cases of insanity. Petitioners for places in Beauport, for example, would frequently be told, after diligently submitting the required documents regarding a specific case of insanity: "In consequence of [the patient's] malady appearing incurable ... I am unable to recommend to His Excellency her admission into the Lunatic Asylum on the footing of a Government Patient. The legislative grant for the support and care of the insane within [the province] being limited, the Executive is compelled to exclude incurable cases, and to reserve the funds disposable for this object for the treatment of cases which offer some chance of cure."[53] This change in asylum policy effectively eliminated asylum committal as an option for a large number of families or communities. The same effect resulted when a financial crisis at the Toronto Asylum caused its commissioners to temporarily prohibit the admission of pauper patients.

The ordeal of petitioning for asylum committal in the face of volatile state policies is particularly well documented in the case of François Blanc. In the opinion of his family, Blanc, a journeyman near Montreal, had become insane. In early June 1853 Blanc's family physician, Dr Paquin, organized a petition for committal, alerting the provincial secretary of his circumstances. "The insane man is in dire poverty with a large family. His wife is in a miserable state, and all their relatives are poor. I address these words to you for the sake of the parish. If there is any way to take her into the asylum, oh! please try to do it. You will never have done a greater service to a family in distress."[54]

Two weeks later Dr Paquin wrote an angry letter to the government expressing his frustration that his petition had not yet been answered and emphasizing again the dire circumstances of his patient's family. This second letter drew a quick response from the government, which stated that there were many petitions similar to Dr Paquin's. Moreover, it was necessary to find accommodation for the large number of lunatics confined in the local jails of the province before individual applications such as his could be considered. Paquin was asked to provide a more detailed report on the specific nature of his patient's madness, including his symptoms and the duration of the disease, while he waited for a response to his petition.

On 4 July Paquin submitted a lengthy report on the medical history of his patient, highlighting the serious long-term debilitating nature of Blanc's mental and physical state. A month and a half later, the government responded that since Dr Paquin's report had indicated that Blanc's insanity was "completely incurable," this diagnosis precluded his admission to the Beauport Asylum. After two and a half months of Paquin's petitioning, the application was summarily rejected.[55]

On occasion, the persistence of the family and community in the petition process could triumph over the official government policies. Dr E.W. Carter, for example, was told that there was no room in the asylum for one of his patients because her condition was considered to be incurable. Carter responded that the patient's husband was leaving for Quebec to "seek a personal interview" with the provincial secretary on the matter. He added that he disagreed with the government's conclusion that his patient was an incurable case. "Certainly ... there is a chance of her recovery," he argued, "under proper treatment in the asylum." In this instance, persistence paid off, and the government admitted the patient for a probationary period of six months, after which she was to be sent back home "should her case prove incurable."[56]

On other occasions, the state appeared to override its own official policies on asylum committal to make "exceptions." Joseph

Dupont, an elderly man, petitioned the government for the committal of his forty-nine-year-old son whom he described as idiotic and epileptic from birth. Dupont relied on begging in the streets of Montreal to support himself and his son. The provincial secretary responded that Dupont's son was decidedly incurable and would not normally be admitted as a government patient. He added, however, that given the particularly unfortunate circumstances of the Dupont's case the government would make an exception in his favour.[57] These "provisional" and "exceptional" examples of admission to the asylum could make a great difference to the circumstances of individual families and communities, but such cases were rare. Their exceptional nature serves as a reminder of the power and authority of the state over the fate of the petitioner.

In Quebec, the power of asylum and state officials to determine asylum admissions was also exerted in more direct ways. The proprietors of the Beauport Asylum, especially during its first two decades, often themselves wrote petitions for committal on behalf of residents of the province whom they deemed worthy of asylum treatment. They also supplied a large number of the medical certificates to support other petitions for committal. With limited asylum accommodation in Quebec, the collusion between medical and political power in such cases was completely transparent. The Beauport proprietors frequently wrote or endorsed petitions assuring the government that a patient's cure was likely under proper treatment within their asylum. Once they received the sanction of the province's leading psychiatric voices, these petitions were guaranteed immediate success. Joseph Morrin, for example, certified one petition in which he recommended that the patient be "removed as soon as possible where she will in all probability soon recover."[58] In other petitions, Morrin specifically linked his petitions for committal to the government's decision to implement a "system of preferring to older cases ... those offering a better chance of cure." These petitions were often certified by co-proprietor James Douglas.[59] The third proprietor, Charles Frémont, similarly issued frequent petitions assuring the provincial secretary of the curable nature of a patient's insanity.[60]

This tendency of Beauport's proprietors to involve themselves in filling their own asylum with patients they judged to be curable could be seen as an effort to ensure that their institution functioned in a manner consistent with mid-nineteenth-century alienist medical principles. But the Beauport proprietors did not restrict their involvement to curable cases. Late in the year 1853, for instance, during a period in which only curable cases were officially being committed to the asylum, Frémont wrote a medical certificate endorsing the admission of Lucie Gerard, a young woman who he hoped would benefit from asylum treatment. Yet Frémont made no mention of her chances of cure. Moreover, in the same petition, Gerard's father noted that his daughter had been insane for three years, a condition he attributed to her epilepsy, which had plagued her for nine years. According to prevailing therapeutic ideas, this was not a hopeful case. Nevertheless, Gerard was granted admission to the asylum.[61] During the same period, several patients who displayed signs of mental aberration similar to or more hopeful than that of Lucie Gerard were denied admission by the government on the grounds that the asylum was restricted to curable cases.[62] In other instances also, the Beauport proprietors successfully petitioned for the admission of patients for whom they held out little hope of recovery.[63] This inconsistency suggests that the Beauport proprietors' decisions on committals were governed by considerations that went beyond prevailing medical ideas on insanity.

In some instances, such preferential treatment was quite obvious. In one petition, Charles Frémont framed his support for a petition in this way: "The applicant is the mother of a young epileptic girl who became insane from a disorganization of intellect. The poor woman is very respectible and is worthy of rescue. She has supported the young girl for many years by procuring for her nursing care, but things have become so much worse for her that both mother and daughter are on the verge of misery ... I do not hesitate to recommend her [for admission] instantly." This petition reads much like many others from various communities of the province. But the status of the medical proprietor guaranteed that this request for committal would be quickly sanctioned by the state.[64]

Others in positions of social and political power were also able to use their influence to affect the fate of a petition for committal. Such manipulation is clearly exemplified by the case of Pierre Leclaire, a farmer from the district of Montreal, who petitioned for the committal of his three brothers. Leclaire claimed that his brothers (aged forty-four, forty-six, and forty-eight) were all idiots, incapable of working or taking care of themselves. He was particularly concerned about the effect of their dirty and vulgar habits on his six children and added that his caring for them for over nine years had placed an immense financial burden on his family.

Of particular note in this petition was a short covering letter written by MPP Augustin-Norbert Morin requesting the attention of the provincial secretary in the matter. On the same day that the petition was sent, the provincial secretary replied that there was no room at the asylum but that the three men would be placed on the waiting list. Four weeks passed with no further response from the government. Dissatisfied with the progress of the petition, Morin again wrote to the provincial secretary (whom he addressed as "My dear Parent") explaining that Pierre Leclaire had been offered money to vote against him in the last elections. Leclaire had refused the bribe on the understanding that Morin would get his brothers into the Beauport Asylum. Morin urged the government to do what it could to expedite Leclaire's petition. The same day that Morin issued his renewed request, the government sanctioned the admission of all three brothers to the asylum.[65]

In evaluating the issue of social and political influence on petitions for committal, it is helpful to consider the analyses of medical historians Charles Rosenberg and Morris Vogel on the development of the hospital in nineteenth-century United States. Rosenberg notes that "in most cases, voluntary hospital admission reflected the patient's place in a network of deference and social relationships." In some institutions, this was made manifest through hospital "subscription," a process whereby "individual philanthropists" paid for the control of a certain number of inpatient beds and outpatient services. Under this system, poor individuals who needed the services of the hospital were obliged to present a signed certificate from a subscriber in order to gain admission to the hospital. Rosenberg argues that "such personal control of access to hospital beds embodied in a concrete way the ties between client and patron fundamental to a deferential and ordered society; the hospital was meant to implement, not supplant such ties."[66]

Although the Beauport Asylum was a different kind of institution and operated in a different social context, it handled admissions of pauper patients in ways similar to that of the mid-nineteenth-century American hospital. Owned and operated by three members of the elite in the socio-medical sphere of Quebec City,[67] and established in relationship with the state as a predominantly charitable institution, the Beauport Asylum embodied the values of a society characterized by social and economic inequality. Petitioning for committal to the lunatic asylum initiated a process in which the deference of the petitioner was made immediately manifest by his or her requests for help from local authority figures (the justice of the peace, the local priest, or the local physician) and from those in higher positions of power (the provincial secretary, the commissioners and the owners of the asylum). In making the decision to commit, individual families and communities were forced to work their way through an intricate hierarchical web of formal and informal social relations. Under these circumstances, the endorsement of a prominent politician or religious figure could be of enormous benefit to the prospects of an ordinary petition for committal. But, as this case involving MP Morin suggests, such an endorsement was unlikely to be secured without some reciprocal obligation on the part of the petitioner.

The complex interplay of social, economic, and political relations set in motion by a petition for committal to the lunatic asylum is strikingly revealed through an examination of the unusual career of Jean-Baptiste Zacharie Bolduc. After being ordained a priest in Quebec in 1841, Bolduc immediately set out on a year-long journey by ship around Cape Horn to the Columbia River, where he helped establish a mission. Nine years later, he returned to Quebec and became the parish priest for St Roche de Quebec and the chaplain for both the Beauport Lunatic Asylum and the Quebec Marine and Emigrant Hospital.[68]

In his role as chaplain to the Beauport Asylum, Bolduc actively involved himself in the affairs of the institution, gaining the confidence of the Beauport proprietors and the government. Within a few years he had become very influential in the process of patient selection for the asylum, being personally responsible for a large percentage of admissions. In 1857 alone, he petitioned for the admission of fifty-one patients. As was the case with the Beauport proprietors, all of the petitions that Bolduc either wrote or endorsed received the sanction of the state. In many instances, the medical certification accompanying Bolduc's petitions were made out by Douglas, Frémont, or Morrin.

Bolduc's influence at the asylum was gained in part through the close relationship that he forged with the assistant provincial secretary, Etienne Parent. The requests for patient admission that Bolduc submitted to Parent were usually informal and friendly. He often began his petitions with a light commentary on his habit of inconveniencing the provincial secretary with his requests. Yet his willingness and his ability to take on many of the administrative aspects of patient committal contributed to his popularity among asylum officials. In many cases, when petitioning to Parent, Bolduc noted that, should his petition be granted, he would handle all of the paper work involved in the committal procedure. He often assured the secretary: "There is no need for you to notify anyone if you will be so kind a to grant my request."[69] This assurance meant that Bolduc himself would serve as the main correspondent between the asylum and the family or community petitioning for asylum committal. He also frequently filled out the questionnaires on the medical history of prospective asylum patients (a task usually performed by individual families and community leaders) and forwarded them to one of the asylum proprietors.[70] This work saved both the government and the proprietors considerable time, and both parties seemed quite willing to devolve these administrative duties to him. Bolduc's responsibilities also greatly expedited the process of committal for patients who fell under his sphere of influence. In this process, Bolduc's word on the mental state and financial circumstances of the patients he sent to the asylum was unquestioned. Eventually a letter of introduction by Bolduc was all that was needed to ensure immediate sanction for a committal. The supporting documents could follow.

Bolduc's acquisition of responsibility and power at Beauport was also due in part to his creative suggestions for accommodating the ever-pressing demand for beds. One of his ideas, which became unofficial policy, evolved out of the government's resistance to accommodate patients for whom Bolduc had petitioned during periods of serious overcrowding at Beauport. In 1856 Bolduc petitioned to the government for the committal to the Quebec General Hospital of a servant named Jane Thomas, who had become insane. The government responded that the state allocation for pauper patients at the Beauport Asylum was at its absolute limit. Bolduc replied that the Sisters at the Quebec General Hospital were willing to take on the care of one of the many docile incurable Beauport patients in exchange a place for Thomas at the asylum. His suggestion was accepted, and the plan was repeated in similar periods of difficulty.[71] On another occasion, Bolduc urged the government to spend $100 to send two sisters, who had recently regained their sanity after a three-year stay at Beauport, back to their family in Ireland. He was of the opinion that the "destitute condition" of the sisters "on their arrival in Canada was the primary cause of their insanity," and that if released from the asylum they would shortly be in need of treatment again. He noted that the sisters themselves had expressed to him their desire to be with their family in Ireland. The government agreed with Bolduc, charging the fees of the sisters' voyage "against the appropriation for the support of the insane" in Quebec.[72]

Bolduc's position at Beauport gave him an insight into asylum policy that he used to acquire accommodation for those he thought in need. He often accompanied his requests for committal with up-to-date statistics on the current and projected patient population at the asylum. This foresight enabled Bolduc to prove to the government that when he petitioned there was in fact room on the pauper list for "his" patients. His ready access to statistics on discharges and deaths at the asylum enabled him frequently to issue "group petitions" requesting the admission of two, three, and sometimes four patients at once. In one request, for example, Bolduc asked for the admission of four people, stating that, "The number of patients has fallen from 382 to 372, and the commissioners' visit at the end of the month will certainly reduce it again by eight or ten. There will be room to accommodate all my requests in the course of this year, I'm sure."[73] Bolduc's knowledge of asylum population statistics and government policy also permitted him to capitalize on periods when more beds were coming available. In a confidential letter to the provincial secretary, for example, he expressed his delight about an impending increase in the allocation of funds for the care of pauper lunatics at Beauport: : "The secretary of the asylum commission told me this morning that you had new funds at your disposal for the asylum in question. Now, you cannot imagine what a joy this news was to me. I have lunatics who were just waiting for this. I will therefore submit to you my requests. There is space to receive up to about 400 patients."[74]

Although most of Bolduc's petitions for committal were on behalf of his own parishioners in St Roches de Quebec, he also petitioned for the accommodation of patients from Quebec City, Montreal, and outlying parishes as well. Much of his knowledge of patients beyond his own parish seems to have come from his correspondence with other priests. Bolduc also visited the homes of patients who had been discharged from the asylum as cured or recovered to check on their progress. Many of his requests were for the readmission of former patients who he believed had relapsed into insanity.[75] He also visited many families to verify the condition of a prospective asylum patient.

In cases of acute illness, or when patients' presence in their homes constituted an immediate threat to their family or a risk to themselves, Bolduc often quickly arranged their committal to the asylum under his own financial responsibility. He then requested that the government retroactively grant the patient "government," or "pauper" status from the date of the original committal. In the case of a woman he considered to be furiously insane, for example, he noted: "If she doesn't become a bit more manageable, I shall be obliged to send her to the asylum without waiting for a response to my petition. I would therefore be infinitely obliged if you would date her admission from this day should the need arise." Bolduc admitted the woman the same day, and the government later approved the petition, establishing her pauper status from the day Bolduc had requested.[76] In another case, Bolduc petitioned that two women he found wandering the streets of Quebec in a wretched state be given government patient status. He admitted them in anticipation of the government's sanction, and asked that "their government patient status be invoked retroactively."[77]

Like the Beauport proprietors, Bolduc often stressed the potential curability of many of the patients for whom he requested asylum committal. In such instances, he usually noted that the Beauport proprietors concurred with his promising assessment of the case. But Bolduc often used his influence to secure places in the asylum for other than merely medical reasons. He sometimes requested the admission of "less curable" cases of insanity as a part of a group petition in which he argued that the other patients on his list showed great promise of immediate cure. In one such petition, he noted that one of his asylum candidates had a form of insanity that was very curable. The other, he admitted, "does not promise as rapid a cure, but nevertheless cannot be considered incurable." In another petition, Bolduc paired a curable case with one that was "incurable, without a doubt." He argued that the case nevertheless demanded the compassion of the state, as the patient was idiotic and would likely die of cold or hunger if left unattended.[78] In several instances, Bolduc petitioned in order to provide some refuge and care for patients who he anticipated would not live long at the asylum.[79]

It is obvious that Bolduc considered a large number of those for whom he petitioned to be socially deserving rather than medically appropriate candidates for the asylum. Yet the moral universe through which he filtered requests for asylum committal did have clear boundaries. In 1857 the provincial secretary asked Bolduc's personal opinion about a petition sent by L.M. Brassard, the parish priest of St Roche de l'Archange, for the committal of two patients. Brassard had apparently mentioned the tacit support of Bolduc in his application. Bolduc responded that Brassard had asked him to help in the process of creating the petition but that he had restricted himself to explaining to Brassard the basic application procedure. In Bolduc's opinion. "Both these patients are incurable ... and their parents appear to want to get rid of them any way they can. Judging by the letter that was written to me, I would not be inclined to react in the same way that I have in many other cases. I have always tried to choose the best cases when I make my requests. If I heeded all those who have asked me to write to you, there would now be more than 600 patients [at the asylum], almost all incurable.[80]

He reassured the provincial secretary that he chose only the "best" cases when making applications for committal, patients for whom cure as possible or for whom no family support was available. When he saw families shirking their responsibilities towards their insane dependents, he considered them undeserving of asylum privileges. Brassard's petition and Bolduc's response highlight the Beauport Asylum chaplain's position of power. As he was responsible for a large percentage of admissions at the asylum on the basis of his own sense of deserving and undeserving candidates, Bolduc's opinion could also have a decisive effect on the fate of other requests for committal. It was clear that families whose petitions did not fall under the chaplin's sphere of influence or did not meet with his favour were less likely to be successful.[81]

Although Bolduc's career was unique, it illustrates the extent to which the process of petitioning for asylum committal in Quebec was dependent upon successful negotiation with those in positions of power at the asylum and state levels. A range of asylum, state, and political officials, along with local legal, religious, and medical authorities, exercised varying degrees of influence over the process of committing people to the asylum as pauper patients. This influence could be felt indirectly, as an effect of changing asylum policy, or more directly, as the expression of political, medical, or religious interests. Individual families certainly used the asylum as a means to help them deal with problems associated with family members considered to be insane. But the road to committal was largely determined by forces over which they had only limited control.

A parallel process of asylum committal in Ontario provided similar challenges for the majority of petitioners to the Toronto Asylum. While medical authority held more sway in Ontario (three medical certificates of insanity were required rather than only one, as required in Quebec), a patient's inability to pay for asylum care in whole or in part needed to be confirmed by the authority of a local justice of the peace or minister or priest, in order for government/pauper status to be considered.

The politics of committal worked differently in Ontario than in Quebec. A sense of this difference can be found in the correspondence between the Toronto Asylum superintendent, Joseph Workman, and the clerk of the peace for Perth county, J.J. Linton. In a candid letter to Linton, Workman vented his frustration about the pressures that accompanied the flood of applications for committal to the Toronto Asylum:

I am *distressed*. Every mail brings me one – two – three urgent letters. Every two or three days some member of parliament presents himself or his written compliments – modestly claiming for some of his constituents the first vacant bed – regardless whether the case is that of some idiot – or long hopeless lunatic – just admit *this* case and confer a favour on the great MPP – or if you do not, look out. Every form of pressure that can be devised is brought to bear on me to induce me to do impossibilities – or to prostitute my function to the purposes of favouritism. I have resolved to withstand *all* and to adhere to the strict rule of right. I can only do the best this house enables me to effect – for a portion of the insane – and I must do this according to my own careful judgement. Have you ever asked your county member what became of the £25,000 voted by parliament in May 1855 to complete this asylum? The insane wretches now rotting in our gaols demand a reply.[82]

Workman's comments indicate that politics and power certainly had as much to do with the process of asylum committal in Ontario as they did in Quebec. It appears however, that Workman considered the exercise of patronage and "favouritism" in asylum admissions to be completely antithetical to his vision of asylum development. He was eloquent on the subject: "Every influence that can be evoked is directed towards securing admissions as *special* favours – and all my firmness (or obstinacy) is required to enable me to withstand these unjust importunities." Workman had fought for, and been granted, the state authority to prioritize admissions according to his philosophy of asylum medicine and treatment. He made his position clear: "As I have always made it my rule to admit the most urgent cases, and those most likely to be benefited, it follows that the outside pressure is exerted in behalf of cases of slightest claim."[83]

Workman's strict policy of admitting only patients who, according to his diagnostic principles, qualified as curable cases of insanity, significantly impeded the success of many petitions for committal based on non-medical grounds. With his power of medical discretion, Workman effectively thwarted the success of many petitions requesting institutionalization for social, economic, and medical reasons that he considered to be "unjust."

Despite Workman's adherence to the "strict rule of right," he was forced to accept a number of patients from the local jails of the province and from elsewhere who were not, in his view, genuine asylum patients amenable to moral treatment. He clung firmly to the principles of his therapeutic outlook on asylum policy. But the interests of the state and those of individuals at the local level who were also stakeholders in the complex relationships affecting the development of the asylum made his position difficult to maintain.

In both provinces, this interplay of interests representing different socio-economic and cultural outlooks needs to be taken into account when attempting to form a comprehensive picture of the provinces' responses to insanity in the nineteenth century. Although, as we have seen, the specific needs and strategies of families and communities played an important role in the process of asylum development, their activities, which reflected their particular set of perspectives on insanity and the asylum, were constrained by the competing and often conflicting perspectives of state and asylum officials, who exercised greater power.

5 Criminal Insanity: The Creation and Dissolution of a Psychiatric Disorder

The brief attempt to medicalize criminal insanity in nineteenth-century Ontario and Quebec highlights the complex interaction of community, state, and psychiatric interests in the process of asylum development. This chapter explores the historical circumstances that led to criminal insanity's classification as a distinct disease entity. The Kingston Penitentiary and the Rockwood Criminal Lunatic Asylum, became the settings for a series of debates and critical incidents focusing on criminal insanity.[1]

In the early years of the century, criminal lunatics were not seen as a social problem of major concern. By mid-century, however, a crisis had emerged in the Kingston Penitentiary over a perceived epidemic of criminal insanity. In an era of emerging institutional responses to various forms of social deviancy, a lively and protracted debate arose over what constituted the most appropriate institutional setting for criminal lunatics. Increasingly thought of as a separate category, criminal lunatics were considered fit subjects for neither the therapeutic treatment of the insane asylum nor the reformatory regimen of the penitentiary. By 1855 the prevailing perception among professional experts was that criminal lunacy was really a medical disorder for which separate institutional provision was needed. For a short period, criminal insanity was "framed" medically.[2] The resolution of this debate in favour of a distinct medical conceptualization of criminal insanity led to the establishment of the Rockwood Criminal Lunatic Asylum in 1855. For the next thirteen years John Palmer Litchfield, medical superintendent of the Rockwood Asylum, attempted to diagnose and then treat the criminally insane. Yet even as the new medical experiment in the treatment of criminal insanity was underway, the altering demands of state officials and of the public steadily chipped away at the medical structure that had been consolidating around the criminally insane. The development of Litchfield's own understanding of the etiology of criminal insanity further contributed to this change in perspective. By the time of Litchfield's death in 1868, the perception of criminal lunacy as a separate medical problem in need of a medical institutional solution had virtually disappeared. Although it had been medically framed for over a decade, criminal insanity was not successfully "medicalized" in Canada before the close of the century.

The treatment of criminal insanity in an asylum setting was established upon a fragile consensus of opinion among professionals from elite psychiatric, legal, medical, and state circles in colonial Canada. As the political, economic, and social circumstances in which this consensus had been reached were altered and other views on criminal insanity came to dominate, the therapeutic response to criminal insanity was hastily rejected and remained so well into the twentieth century.

Violations of the law by criminal lunatics in nineteenth-century Quebec and Ontario included arson, assault and battery, and murder. Most offenders were formally charged and tried for their crimes. If, during their trials, they were found to be insane, they were deemed not responsible for their criminal acts. In the words of Attorney General William Draper, "The fact of insanity existing at the time of the commission of any act for which a party is indictable will wholly excuse him from the penal consequences attached to the act."[3] Criminal lunatics also included prisoners found to be unable to stand trial due to their insanity and inmates who manifested symptoms of insanity after conviction.[4]

Before the creation of provisional or temporary lunatic asylums in British North America, criminals who were acquitted of responsibility for their crimes on the grounds of insanity were generally kept in district or local jails and tended to by local physicians.[5] After the temporary asylums were opened (in 1839 in Lower Canada, and

1841 in Upper Canada) occasional transfers from local jails to the provisional asylum were initiated by a county clerk of the peace, a local sheriff, or the judge of a particular trial.[6]

After initial charges were laid against them, insane criminals often experienced protracted stays in these jails waiting for the local assizes, to arrive try their cases following their routine of scheduled stops. Upon a verdict of not guilty by reason of insanity, an insane criminal was further detained in jail while a position in the provisional asylum was sought.[7] Further delays in the transfer of criminal lunatics to the provisional asylums might be occasioned by the overcrowding of the new proto-institutions. As with the "ordinary insane," the backlog of applicants to the temporary asylums meant that criminal lunatics were confined for long periods in district jails. Before mid-century, the numbers of criminally insane were small, and criminal insanity had generated little attention as a social issue.

A developing crisis in social organization at the Kingston Penitentiary focused greater attention on the subject of criminal insanity, however. This focus in turn altered perceptions among legal, medical, and psychiatric authorities about insane criminals and the best means to their reform. Initially, provision for the criminally insane at the Kingston Penitentiary tended to mirror their treatment in local jails. Until 1850 there was a noticeable absence of criminal lunatics in reports by James Sampson, the penitentiary surgeon. Between 1836, when the penitentiary opened, and 1849, there were only five entries in his medical records concerning convicts suffering from "mental derangement." Of those, three were removed to the temporary lunatic asylum in Toronto, one was transferred to the Beauport Lunatic Asylum near Quebec, and the last committed suicide in the penitentiary.[8]

This situation changed dramatically within a few years. In 1849 Sampson pointed out to the inspectors of the penitentiary that there were then "three male and two female Convicts labouring under various forms of mental derangement" in the penitentiary. The surgeon expressed his concern that the penitentiary had "no means of carrying on the proper *moral management* of these subjects, according to the specific character of each," and he advised the inspectors that the five criminal lunatics would be best placed in "an Asylum where already all the necessary appliances are in the hands of persons trained in the management of this affliction in all its forms."[9] By 1850 the list of insane convicts had grown to nine,

Table 2   Return of Insane Convicts in the Kingston Penitentiary during the Year 1850

Name	Age	Disease	Remarks
James Jackson	43	Dementia	From Montreal. Is in general harmless. In hospital at large.
John Carlisle	39	Mania	In hospital under confinement. Vicious, noisy and dangerous.
Elizabeth Keith	58	Mania	In hospital under confinement.
Paul Jones	41	Mania	Very mischievous, vicious and noisy. Confined to cell.
Michael Walther	24	Mania	Very mischievous. Confined to cell.
Henry Carter	31	Mania	Suicidal and homicidal periodically.
John Giles	30	Mania	
Charles Fenton	50	Unsound Mind	Periodical delusions (harmless)
James Proudfoot	?	Mania	From Montreal. Removed from work crew 1 December 1850. Is of unsound mind and dangerous

Source: Table compiled from information from NA, Records of the Provincial Secretary, Canada West, RG5 C1, file 435, 1850; and *JLAUC*, Report of the Penitentiary Physician, 1 October 1851.

not counting one female convict of "unsound mind," who had been sent to the recently opened permanent Toronto Provincial Asylum, and one male convict suffering from "mental delusions," who had been released when his prison term had expired.[10] (See Table 2.)

Among the officers of the penitentiary, there were competing explanations for the growing incidence of insanity in the inmate population. According to the penitentiary's Board of Inspectors, "mental aberration" in the prison had "not originated from the discipline, or any causes existing within the Penitentiary itself." The board did, however, suggest that "the tendency and predisposition to *dementia* and insanity [might], in some degree, have been developed from confinement in a situation where the individuals were of necessity deprived of old associations and accustomed habits." In one case, they noted, an inmate tried for murder was found to be insane at the time of his criminal act. After being brought to the penitentiary, his hallucinations worsened to the point where his reason was "irrevocably lost." In the inspectors' opinion, the other insane convicts on Sampson's list "were persons of naturally weak mind, subject to delusion, and therefore, readily plunging into error and crime – a class of individuals that may be said to be affected with incipient mania before its actual manifestations." Their contention was clear. Convict insanity was not primarily the result of the penitentiary environment.[11]

Sampson's opinion on the increasing numbers of insane convicts differed significantly from that of the penitentiary inspectors. The surgeon argued that out of twenty-four cases of insanity "which from time to time appeared in the prison, sixteen were as far as could be ascertained, first manifested therein." Therefore, he asserted, the "invasion of [the] intellectual disorders [of those sixteen] was induced by a combination of causes incidental to their imprisonment." To Sampson, "the [removal of] the existing causes of mental as well as bodily derangements, is ... the first indication of successful treatment" in a penal institution. The increase in criminal insanity was thus, in his view, a symptom of a defective institution.[12]

The differing explanations of Sampson and the Board of Commissioners for the rise in insanity among the prison convicts were an aspect of a more fundamental conflict over the proper management of the penitentiary. For most of the 1840s the warden, Henry Smith, appeared to dominate the administrative affairs of the penitentiary. He also condoned the "extensive use of corporal punishment" on the convicts. Public criticism of Smith's regime and internal fighting between Sampson and the Board of Inspectors led to the formation of a royal commission in 1848 on the "conduct, economy, system of discipline and management, pursued" in the penitentiary. The ensuing investigation uncovered conclusive evidence of "brutal and excessive punishment of prisoners." Although Sampson was never explicit about the exact causes of insanity "incidental to imprisonment" that he had in mind, there can be little doubt that he viewed the disciplinary excesses uncovered by the royal commission as a contributing factor in the mental deterioration of certain convicts.[13]

Evidence gathered from the royal commission further points to conflict between the surgeon and the warden over the corporal punishment meted out to the inmates. The commission's investigators discovered, for example, that during an eight-year period, prisoner Paul Stephenson "was ordered 1002 lashes of the cats, and 216 of the raw hide; but 36 lashes of the cats having been stopped by the Surgeon [who diagnosed him as insane], the whole number of lashes inflicted on him has been 1182." They concluded that Stephenson's punishments "greatly aggravated his predisposition to insanity." Stephenson was one of several insane convicts whose punishment histories resulted in charges being laid against the warden for "goading ... by excessive punishment ... into a state of insanity, or in aggravating the malady under which [the prisoners] laboured."[14] Smith's free use of corporal punishment to maintain discipline and order in the penitentiary was clearly opposed by Sampson's view that this same system of physical coercion was contributing to the rise in insanity among the convict population. However, whether these prisoners were "diabolical beings,"as Smith believed, or "mentally deranged,"as Sampson saw them, neither warden nor surgeon considered the penitentiary a suitable place for their incarceration.

Support for this common opinion was reflected in the Royal Commission's passage of An Act for the Better Management of the Provincial Penitentiary on 1 August 1851. Partly on the basis of Sampson's repeated warnings about the growing crisis of criminal lunacy in the penitentiary, this new legislation allowed for "the removal, under certain conditions," of criminal lunatics from the penitentiary to the recently established Provincial Lunatic Asylum in Toronto.[15] A Board of Physicians was also appointed by the government to report on cases of insanity arising in the penitentiary.[16] The act enabled Sampson to send seven insane convicts to the Toronto Provincial Lunatic Asylum in the fall of 1851, a decision which, according to the surgeon, "tended to remove a considerable source of anxiety from the minds of those concerned in their care, as well as to improve the situation, and meliorate the condition of the sufferers."[17] Section Four of An Act to Authorize the Confinement of Lunatics in Cases Where Their Being at Large May Be Dangerous to the Public passed four weeks later on 30 August 1851, and authorized the removal of insane persons from "any prison, or other place of confinement" to the "public Lunatic Asylum, or other proper receptacle for insane persons."[18]

The departure of the seven criminal lunatics along Lake Ontario from the Kingston Penitentiary reassured Surgeon Sampson that his patients of unsound mind were heading to the proper institution of moral management. However, their transfer to the Toronto Provincial Asylum aroused great concern in its superintendent, John Scott. Scott's objections were threefold. First, he was of the opinion that in some cases the professed insanity of the convicts was "very doubtful." He argued that the prisoners often feigned madness, "hoping thus to escape the horrors of a prison, and enjoy the comparative comfort and freedom of a Lunatic Asylum." Second, he argued that "in the erection of [the Toronto Provincial Lunatic Asylum], it was probably never considered that such a class should be sent here, and hence no provision was made for their security against escape." His third concern centred on the question of whether these newly arrived criminal lunatics were to have "free and unrestricted intercourse with the other patients."[19] Scott's reservations in regard to the care of the criminally insane indicate that this new category of patients would fit awkwardly within the structure of treatment embodied in the newly established Toronto Provincial Lunatic Asylum.

By the time Joseph Workman, the newly appointed replacement of Superintendent Scott, penned his first annual report for the Toronto Asylum in 1853, reaction to the arrival of criminal lunatics from the Provincial Penitentiary and from local jails had turned to outrage. In Workman's view:

An evil of inconceivable magnitude, and distressing results, in the working and present condition of this Institution has been the introduction into it of Criminal Lunatics from the Provincial Penitentiary, and the County Gaol. It is an outrage against public benevolence, and an indignity to human affliction, to cast into the same house of refuge with the harmless, kind-hearted and truthful victims of ordinary insanity, those *moral monsters*, which nature sometimes seems to have formed, for the purpose of teaching us the inestimable value of the constitution with which the species has been blessed.[20]

Like Scott, Workman also suggested that in "several cases" the criminal lunatics who had arrived at the Toronto Asylum were "imposters" who caused "more moral detriment, to both Patients and Keepers than twenty real mad-men." As long as "the law which orders the transmission to the Asylum of Penitentiary and Jail patients … continues to exist," concluded Workman, "it must be impossible to preserve that salutary discipline and mild management, which are indispensable to the successful operation of the institution." In Workman's opinion, it was imperative that "more appropriate provision" be made by the provincial government "for the disposal of [this] class of patients."[21] Workman's anger over the arrival of criminal lunatics was further fuelled by his inability to segregate these unwanted patients from the ordinary insane. In 1853 only three wards of the Toronto Asylum had been completed. As Workman was a strong proponent of classification according to the principles of moral therapy, he considered the addition of yet another category of lunatics an "outrage" to the theory and practice of asylum medicine.

From the first implementation of the amended Penitentiary Act, it was obvious that Workman would not tolerate the presence in his institution of the majority of criminal lunatics sent from Kingston. He made his own assessment of incoming criminal lunatics on the basis of their personal background, their social behaviour in the asylum, and the reason they had been convicted. These three criteria decided how long they would remain in his institution. Workman was willing to provide asylum treatment for those whose crimes were slight – for example mild instances of forgery, or theft – and whose behaviour in the asylum posed little challenge to institutional discipline.[22] He also seemed willing to care for those who came from settings that may have contributed to the onset of their insanity. For example, Allen Brown, who was admitted to the asylum on 13 May 1853 had been charged with "assault and threatening to kill his mother." Yet Workman noted that Brown arrived at the asylum "in a deplorable condition, both of body and mind," a condition largely due to a combination of "hardship, defective diet, and harsh paternal controul." The boy's responsibility for his crime (and his insanity), was in Workman's view mitigated by the social context within which his behaviour had taken place.

In a more dramatic example, Elizabeth Pearson arrived at the Toronto Asylum on 18 April 1853 having killed her two children in an "instantaneous, or impulsive" moment of insanity. From Pearson's own accounts, Workman learned that she had been "badly treated by her husband, and that her object in killing her children was to secure their early admission into heaven, and save them from the sufferings such as she herself had undergone." For Workman, there was a clear connection between the crime and Pearson's sufferings at the hands of her husband. She was thus given refuge at the asylum.[23] What the few criminal lunatics that Workman decided to keep at the Toronto Asylum had in common was their relatively non-disruptive acceptance of institutional order.

But the majority of the prisoners sent from Kingston were in Workman's opinion either "imposters" who "affected" mental alienation as a "device by which to evade the just punishment" of the law, or "depraved and bloodthirsty criminals whose habits of violence [had] become confirmed and [might], even in returning sanity, be held in greatest dread." There would be no place for such disruptive "moral monsters" in an asylum for the "ordinary insane."[24] In order to bypass the workings of the new Penitentiary Act, Workman simply reported that most incoming criminal lunatics had recovered their sanity shortly after arriving at the Toronto Asylum, whereupon he shipped them right back to the penitentiary. Through the medical authority invested in him, Workman in effect revoked the medical status of the criminal lunatics, rendering them criminals proper, once more candidates for the penitentiary.

Two examples of this practice in particular are noted in some detail by Penitentiary Surgeon James Sampson. Michael Mather was sentenced to death for the murder of his father, mother, and sister when he burned down the family home. His sentence was commuted to life imprisonment by the Provincial Penitentiary, as he was considered to have been insane while committing the crime. Sampson argued that Mather displayed ample evidence of his insane condition during his stay at the penitentiary and sent Mather to the Toronto Asylum on 2 December 1851. Workman returned Mather to the penitentiary nine months and three weeks later reporting that he was "of sound mind." In Sampson's view, however, "No improvement has taken place and he has, since his return, been confined to his Cell, in consequence of an evident disposition he evinces to do violence to those who approach him, under the delusion that they are about to take him to the Gallows." A second patient, Alex Rousseau, faced the same sentence for killing a fellow prisoner in the local jail in Three Rivers, Canada East, "under the impression that the victim of his delusion was conspiring with his family to murder him." In 1852 Rousseau was also sent to the Toronto Asylum and was returned by Workman as cured six weeks and two days later. Sampson was convinced that these two patients and several others had "no amelioration of their mental condition" while at the Toronto Asylum and argued that their return to the penitentiary merely reflected Workman's unwillingness to treat the criminally insane.[25]

Sampson was particularly distressed about Rousseau's case because the convict patient spoke only French. The surgeon suggested that the fact that Rousseau's hallucinations at the Toronto Asylum were "expressed in his own language" and may not have been understood by the medical and non-medical staff would have rendered treatment ineffectual. Sampson noted his regret that the Act for the Better Management of the Provincial Penitentiary had not made provision for the transfer of criminal lunatics of French Canadian origin from the Kingston Penitentiary to the Beauport Asylum.[26]

It is evident, however, that during this period the Act for the Confinement of Lunatics was being used to transfer the criminally insane from local jails to the Beauport Asylum. In the winter of 1853, for example, Montreal resident Anne Dupont was convicted of infanticide, having dispatched her newborn child into a privy. Dupont was imprisoned, but was subsequently found to have been insane at the time of her criminal act and was sent to the Beauport Asylum for treatment. A year later Beauport proprietors Morrin and Frémont reported to the provincial secretary that Dupont had fully recovered her sanity. She was therefore removed to the local jail from which she had originally been convicted and released shortly thereafter. Another Montreal resident, Jean Marchand, was charged with horse stealing, but was subsequently found to be insane. Marchand was also transferred to the Beauport Asylum, where, after several months, he was considered by the Beauport proprietors to have recovered his sanity. He was transferred back to the Montreal District Jail and then officially released.[27]

These and other examples indicate that the new law on criminal insanity was used for the removal of the criminally insane in Quebec to the Beauport Asylum. Yet there is no indication that Beauport's asylum superintendents responded to the arrival of the criminally insane with anger or outrage as their counterparts in Ontario had done. This relative absence of indignation can be explained in a number of ways. First, with more out-buildings and greater means of patient classification, the Beauport Asylum probably had more facilities than its counterpart in Toronto for dealing with a class of patients labelled criminally insane. Second, unlike the case in the Toronto Asylum at mid-century, mechanical restraint to deal with behaviour considered violent or unmanageable was still in official use at Beauport. Finally, it is possible that the Beauport proprietors' particular outlook on asylum medicine gave them a more pragmatic view of the presence of criminally insane patients in their asylum.

Although the application of the criminal lunacy laws in Quebec resulted in the relatively uneventful transfer of the criminally insane from local jails to the Beauport Asylum, conflict over this same process continued unabated in Ontario. The forceful appeals of the penitentiary surgeon for "appropriate" moral treatment of the criminally insane, and Workman's refusal to have these patients cared for at the Toronto Asylum, eventually created a mid-century socio-therapeutic crisis. The impasse between the two arguments generated considerable concern among prominent members of Kingston's emerging political, legal, and medical elite. Physicians James Sampson and John Dickson, along with Attorney General and prominent Kingston lawyer John A. Macdonald, were particularly instrumental in promoting a medical solution to the crisis of criminal insanity. Kingston was rising to prominence as a centre of political and medical activity. It was from that context that the eventual resolution to this crisis emerged.

Macdonald's concern with the growing crisis of criminal insanity in the United Canadas was sparked initially by his experience as Attorney General. In this capacity, Macdonald was called upon to advise in several cases of criminal lunacy. Moreover, Macdonald was aware of Superintendent Joseph Workman's complaints "of the evils arising from the reception of insane criminals" at the Toronto Provincial Asylum and he concurred with the superintendent that it was imperative to provide "a separate place of confinement for that class of lunatics."[28]

Macdonald no doubt received further counsel on the need to provide separate facilities for the criminally insane from Drs Sampson and Dickson. In the late 1840s and early 1850s, Sampson and Dickson, along with a few other regular physicians, had gained status in Kingston through their affiliation with the city's fledgling medical institutions and through their medical care of prominent members of the political establishment. The growing prominence of these and other regular practitioners in Kingston was further consolidated by the establishment of the medical department at Queen's University on 6 November 1854. John A.

Macdonald was instrumental in facilitating the intellectual ambitions of the medical elite. He called two founding meetings at his house in early February, at which the physicians chose a medical faculty and decided on course topics to be presented to the trustees of Queen's University. Although his own understanding of criminal lunacy was drawn largely from his legal and political career, Macdonald's close association with a rising group of professional medical men led him to conceptualize criminal insanity as a fundamentally medical problem in need of an institutionalized medical solution.[29]

On 27 February 1855 Macdonald recommended to the provincial secretary that since "that portion of the Provincial Penitentiary at Kingston lately occupied as a military prison has been given up by the military authorities and is now unoccupied, it could be easily fitted up for the reception of the criminal lunatics in the [Provincial] Asylum, now 21 in number, as well as for those at present confined in the several county Gaols of Upper Canada." Macdonald further recommended that "the undivided attention of a medical superintendent [would] be required for the proper treatment" of the criminally insane.[30] A week later Macdonald advised the provincial secretary that John Palmer Litchfield was "a fit and proper person to fill" the position of superintendent of the proposed criminal lunatic asylum at Kingston.[31]

Litchfield was a logical choice for several reasons. Originally from Liverpool, he had come to Canada when applying for the position of medical superintendent of the Toronto Provincial Asylum vacated by John Scott in 1853. The position was ultimately given to Joseph Workman who had been acting as the asylum's temporary medical director. But out of a field of fifty applicants Litchfield was one of six candidates short-listed for the post. Moreover, unlike most of the other applicants, he had decided to settle in Canada despite not being the chosen candidate and established a strong presence in elite social and political circles in Quebec and Ontario.[32] The Governor General made Litchfield's position official six weeks later.[33]

The establishment of the Rockwood Criminal Lunatic Asylum under the superintendency of Litchfield marked the official recognition of a new category of deviancy – criminal insanity.[34] It was hoped that criminal insanity, like other forms of insanity, could be successfully treated within a medical institutional context.

According to asylum inspectors Wolfred Nelson and Andrew Dickson, one of the primary functions of the criminal lunatic asylum would be Litchfield's "scientific treatment" of the criminally insane. A criminal lunatic asylum would provide the opportunity for "a close and critical observation of the phenomena attendant upon aberration of the intellect." Furthermore, "the opportunities thus afforded for the study of these manifestations, both during life and after death, would contribute largely to a correct knowledge of the origin and the source of the diseases, and in a proportional degree to a more or less successful treatment of them."[35] The criminal lunatic asylum was to be a laboratory for the study of the etiology of criminal insanity and of how best to cure various manifestations of the disease. Theoretically, criminal insanity was to be firmly entrenched within a medical/scientific framework. As an institution established for the United Provinces of Canada East and Canada West, the Rockwood Criminal Lunatic Asylum was to provide treatment for the criminally insane of both provinces.

By the mid-1850s, a consensus had emerged among the political, legal, and medical elites: criminal insanity was a specific mental disorder requiring the development of a specialized psychiatric medical science. This consensus was fragile, however, and remained intact, mainly on the theoretical level, for only a short time. In reality, the medical treatment of the criminally insane was conducted from the outset under circumstances completely inconsistent with the theoretical underpinnings of the professional consensus. The gap between theory and practice in the institutional management and treatment of the criminally insane was much wider than that which obtained for the "ordinary" insane in Quebec and Ontario. As the establishment of the Rockwood Criminal Lunatic Asylum gradually defused the crisis created by the conflicts between Sampson and Workman, the government abandoned criminal insanity as a priority. The development of creative strategies for asylum committal at the community level further unravelled the professional consensus on criminal insanity as a particular psychiatric disorder.

While the idea of treating the criminally insane within a medical institutional framework was novel to mid-nineteenth-century Canada, Litchfield did not carry on his work in an intellectual vacuum. During his superintendency at the Walton Asylum near

Liverpool, Litchfield had been exposed to the ideas of British alienists on criminal insanity.[36] He drew upon these intellectual precedents when writing his annual reports for the Rockwood Asylum, citing the work of W.C. Hood, resident medical officer in charge of criminal lunatics in London's Bethlem Hospital at mid-century, and that of prominent English alienist, Sir John Charles Bucknill.[37] While this growing body of literature on the theory and practice of criminal insanity contributed to his understanding of, and dealings with, his insane charges, Litchfield's medical outlook was also informed by his day-to-day treatment of patients and altered by the spatial limitations asylum in which he carried out his work.

Although a new asylum for criminal lunatics was planned and eventually built during Litchfield's superintendentship, initially two separate provisional asylums were established.[38] Female patients were lodged in two structures that were formerly part of the estate of John Cartwright known as the Rockwood Estate. Cartwright's large stone stables were renovated to accommodate twenty-four female patients, and a small stone cottage nearby was later used to house a few more. The "stable-asylum" consisted of twenty single rooms nine feet by five feet each, as well as a wooden addition for four more patients. These rooms "were lighted by ... barred peep-holes, measuring only 18 inches by 12 inches."[39] In 1857 the main building of the Cartwright Estate was purchased by the government and converted by Litchfield into a more permanent asylum for forty female patients.[40]

This accommodation compared favourably with the "wretched state" of asylum provision for the male patients. Male criminal lunatics were at first allotted a separate space in the west wing of the Kingston Penitentiary that had formerly been occupied by military convicts.[41] Due to the increasing numbers of prisoners sent to the penitentiary, however, Litchfield was forced to relocate his criminally insane male charges to the basement of the penitentiary dining hall in 1856. This moist and dismal asylum below ground level was deplored by asylum inspectors as "miserably cramped," and "a sad place for sick persons."[42] The unfortunate state of the male asylum and complaints that it was taking up space needed for ordinary prisoners led to pleas for its relocation.[43] Nevertheless, it was not until 1862 that enough of the new asylum was completed to partially relieve the unsatisfactory conditions. The dining rooms of the new, partially completed Rockwood Asylum were arranged to accommodate some of the patients from the unhealthy penitentiary basement.[44] By the end of 1864, twenty-two male lunatics were removed from the temporary asylum to the east wing of the new Rockwood Asylum, "leaving 48 still in the wretched basement of the Penitentiary." On 24 March 1865, the east wing of the Rockwood Asylum was sufficiently complete to transfer the remaining forty-eight male patients.[45] As for the female patients, it was not until shortly before Litchfield's death in 1868 that they were transferred to the new asylum.

From a therapeutic standpoint, the provisional asylum period was marked predominantly by Litchfield's efforts as a medical practitioner to forestall the steady decline in the physical health of his male patients. Observing that "the patients of the Female Asylum at Rockwood [had] been throughout very healthy," he remarked that the physical health of the male patients had suffered greatly as a result of their poor living conditions in the temporary asylum.[46] Litchfield persistently warned the asylum inspectors that the health and safety of his male patients depended on the speedy completion of the new asylum.[47] In 1862 he attributed the relative wellness of some of the male lunatics to the transfer "of those of the patients who were in a declining state of health" from the temporary asylum in the basement of the penitentiary to "some larger and better ventilated apartments fitted up as convalescent wards in the building in course of erection at Rockwood."[48]

Tuberculosis was the greatest immediate threat to the health of the male patients. Litchfield attributed three of the four patient deaths in 1863 to "pulmonary consumption." In 1864 his postmortem examinations revealed that out of eleven deaths nine were due to "phthisis," seven of these victims being male patients. Asylum inspectors acknowledged that the percentage of tuberculosis deaths in the provisional asylum was much higher than in any of the other Canadian asylums.[49] Litchfield noted that the 9.1 per cent mortality rate for 1864 "was chiefly confined to those patients who had been immured for successive generations in the underground apartments, beneath the dining hall of the Penitentiary."[50] While urging the immediate completion of the new asylum so that his patients could benefit from its "larger and better ventilated apartments," Litchfield made efforts to organize the provisional asylum to serve the medical needs of the male criminal lunatics.[51]

Despite the constraints placed on his practice by the physical conditions of the new Rockwood Criminal Lunatic Asylum, Litchfield gradually developed a distinctive therapeutic outlook on the treatment of criminal insanity. His understanding of the medical needs of his patient population was shaped partly by prevailing modes of medical practice and partly by his own experience of working with the criminally insane. He believed that in order to successfully treat and classify the criminally insane in an asylum it was important to study "minutely the history of every case, the peculiar features of the malady and the temper and disposition of the individual." Such careful observation, he argued, would enable him to acquire the "confidence of the patient" and thus improve the chances of a cure. This combination of close familiarity with the history and habits of the patient and the gradual development of a patient's faith in the superintendent's ability to cure was considered essential to the success of the institutional practice of most mid-nineteenth-century alienists.[52] Litchfield's view was that such orthodox strategy applied equally to all criminal lunatics regardless of the nature of their crimes.

This therapeutic philosophy is exemplified by Litchfield's diagnosis and treatment of Gregory Meighen, a soldier of His Majesty's 17th Regiment, who shot and killed Colonel Sergeant Ryalls during a military parade in Quebec. In an initial interview, Litchfield observed that Meighen demonstrated "confusion of ideas, and dizziness in the head." Furthermore, Meighen stated that "prior to the commission of the crime for which he was tried he had indulged freely in drink, which had the effect of producing great excitement in him." Litchfield next made an investigation into Meighen's medical and psychiatric history by communicating with the surgeon of Meighen's regiment, with some of his former comrades in the Royal Canadian Rifles, and with James Douglas, one of the proprietors of the Beauport Asylum, who had given evidence at Meighen's trial. Douglas assured Litchfield that Meighen had definitely been insane when he committed the murder. Meighen's military comrades informed Litchfield that "he had been subject to delusions" and, perhaps more significantly, that in Ireland Meighen's father occasionally suffered from attacks and was known locally as "mad Meighen." On the basis of this reconstructed history, Litchfield concluded that Meighen suffered from the "hereditary taint of recurring insanity" or "recurrent mania," a condition which, when "excited" by "the use of alcoholic drinks," had predisposed him to murder Colonel Ryalls. After three years under Litchfield's care, the "symptoms of which Meighen complained were removed," and he no longer exhibited "any sign of mental aberration."[53]

Sometimes Litchfield attributed long-term recovery to the removal of the patient from the social circumstances that had originally led to criminal insanity. Treatment of patients in controlled environments away from their home and community social setting of course formed part of the rationale of the lunatic asylum itself. But once a patient had recovered in his asylum, Litchfield also tried to make certain that pre-existing detrimental social influences had been eliminated before the patient was released back into the community. An example of such a case, was his treatment of Robert Davis, a farmer who had become embroiled in a dispute with a neighbouring farmer over the boundary line between their properties. The dispute had escalated to the point where Davis attacked his neighbour and was charged with assault and battery. He was sentenced to five years hard labour in the Kingston Penitentiary. Soon after his arrival in jail, he was deemed insane by the penitentiary surgeon and transferred as a criminal lunatic into Litchfield's care. According to Litchfield, Davis at first "labored under great excitement" in the asylum, manifesting a desire to "quarrel and to assault those about him." He was diagnosed with acute mania. After six months in the criminal lunatic asylum, Litchfield reported that Davis's "state of mental alienation [had] gradually passed away." Nevertheless, as he did not consider Davis to be "a man of strong mind," he warned Abigail, his wife, that if her husband returned to his "former residence" he would be exposed again "to the causes which before produced his mental excitement." After consultation with Litchfield, Abagail Davis decided to move her family to the "western states of the union."[54]

According to Litchfield, only the expert observations of a qualified superintendent could determine when a full recovery from criminal lunacy had actually occurred. His emphasis on the proper timing for the release of recovered criminal lunatic patients is illustrated by the case of Jane Cloverdale. Cloverdale was admitted to the criminal lunatic asylum on 13 July 1863 and diagnosed with puerperal mania, a form of insanity which Litchfield thought had driven her to murder her own newborn child, try to kill another child, and attempt suicide. Litchfield's opinion was that her insanity was brought on by her family's economic distress during her confinement. Fear that her family members would face starvation had induced her to attempt to kill them rather than subjecting them to long-term misery and suffering. Litchfield described her on intake as "very much wasted in person, melancholy and prostrated in mind and so nervous and shrinking that it was with great difficulty she could be got to take any interest in what was passing about her." By December 1864, however, she had improved to the point that her husband, confident that she was sufficiently recovered, petitioned for her release.

In his medical report, Litchfield acknowledged that after several months of care in the asylum Cloverdale had gradually recovered her "bodily health" and become "free from any symptoms of mental aberrations." But she had a history that caused him to express reservations about releasing her before he could be certain of a full recovery:

Her insanity may recur if she is again pregnant. She is 45 years of age and if she was past the turn of life I should have no fear of a recurrence of the insanity. If it does recur she would be melancholy, desponding, suicidal ... Jane Cloverdale after a previous confinement became an inmate of the Toronto Asylum. She was discharged cured from that asylum after a few months treatment in it just as she might be discharged from this asylum were it not for the fact that the same result may follow the same exciting cause. I find also that after one of her confinements she was an inmate of the House of Recovery at Preston Lancashire and that she suffered then from an attack of puerperal mania.

Litchfield decided to postpone her discharge until he could properly test her fitness to "go out into the world." This he did by giving her additional freedom within the asylum, and by gradually bringing her into contact with some local acquaintances of the asylum's matron, Louisa Jane Litchfield. During this interval Litchfield also took the opportunity to suggest to Cloverdale's husband "the precautions which occur to me to guard the patient against the chances of a relapse." As he had done with other patients, Litchfield suggested that, if possible, the Cloverdales "change the locality of [their] residence where everything would remind her of the sad tragedy in which she was an actor." By 12 April 1865, Litchfield decided that Cloverdale had suddessfully passed the probationary period, and recommended her discharge.[55]

Although the initial symptoms of criminally insane patients might have subsided under asylum care, Litchfield nevertheless felt that a permanent or complete recovery was in some cases very unlikely. James Jackson, for example, was charged in 1845 with the murder of a friend in a shooting incident. A commission *de lunatico inquirendo* found that Jackson was suffering from chronic mania brought on by intemperance. He was incarcerated in the Kingston Penitentiary as a criminal lunatic, and then transferred into Litchfield's care in 1855 when the criminal lunatic asylum was opened. The superintendent reported that over a ten-year period Jackson gradually took over responsibility as cook for the asylum. By 1865 he was preparing meals for the 110 male patients under Litchfield's charge and conducting himself with "the utmost regularity" and "cleanliness." Jackson was no longer dangerous, but, according to Litchfield, his delusions persisted and he had an "incessant hankering for drink" – the aggravating cause of his criminal insane act. Litchfield would not risk Jackson's release from the asylum.[56]

As the foregoing examples suggest, towards the end of his career Litchfield came to see criminal lunacy not so much as the *distinct* disease entity it was considered to be a decade earlier, but rather as a peculiar manifestation of ordinary insanity. Relying on traditional alienist diagnostic methods and treatment strategies that emphasized the standard moral therapeutic triumvirate of work, amusement, and religious instruction, Litchfield's treatment of criminal lunatics was virtually indistinguishable from that of his alienist counterparts in asylums for the "ordinary insane" in Quebec and Ontario.

By the 1860s Litchfield had begun to inform asylum inspectors about his views on the similarities between the criminal and the ordinary insane. He described cases of criminal lunatics who had committed murder but who nevertheless responded positively to his careful moral management much as any insane patient might recover. He used these examples in an effort to demonstrate his view that the proper medical classification of the criminally insane "should be founded upon the form and character of the disease, not upon the gravity of the offense committed." In essence, the criminal component of his criminal lunatic patients was largely irrelevant in determining either the form of their treatment or their chances of recovery. He had come to view criminal lunatics as no more potentially dangerous or violent than the ordinary insane and argued that their recovery rate would be greatly improved if they were treated in regular insane asylums in association with the ordinary insane.[57]

By distancing himself from the view that criminal insanity constituted a distinct psychiatric disorder, Litchfield took a clear position in a debate emerging among asylum officials about the architectural principles to be integrated into the new Rockwood Criminal Lunatic Asylum. This debate, which centred on the conflicting opinions of the inspector of prisons, Dr Wolfred Nelson, and Superintendent Joseph Workman, signalled a further breakdown in the fragile consensus on criminal insanity that had been reached in 1855. Shortly before asylum construction began in 1859, Nelson expressed grave concerns about the architectural plans for the new building: "It would appear that the object to be attained and the real nature of this establishment was, at the very threshold lost sight of, that is to be a penal institution; instead of which the whole outline, internal distribution and appliances, convey the idea that this structure is for an ordinary asylum for lunatics, such as one not tainted with crime, but of respectable position, and connected with society by all the ties of affection and family affinities."[58] More specifically, he objected to the "extravagant" scale upon which the design of the new asylum was based. Criminal lunatics, he argued, did not require the conveniences of an asylum for the ordinary insane such as school rooms, a library, large "cells," and spacious grounds. An asylum for criminal lunatics should be "plain and secure with an entire absence of ornament; it could be built cheap and yet as comfortable as need be, and not by its aspect and costly appendances, invite to deceit in order, through crime to obtain a smug and permanent residence, where every want is supplied and as it were officiously attended to, yea, even to pampering and administering to every caprice."[59]

Nelson was willing to stake his reputation "as a medical man" on his belief that the proposal for Rockwood was completely counter to the aims of institutional management of the criminally insane. As far as he was concerned, to lodge the criminally insane in a building whose architectural principles reflected in theory and practice the moral treatment of the ordinary insane was to fundamentally misunderstand the unique character of the criminal lunatic. In the final analysis, the Rockwood Asylum ought in his view to be considered first and foremost a penal institution for patients morally corrupted by their criminal acts. Continuing with the proposed plans for the Rockwood Asylum would "injuriously affect the reputation of the [medical] faculty, and all who are concerned in its construction and management."[60]

Nelson's warnings about the misguided design for the Rockwood construction led the provincial secretary to solicit a second opinion from the superintendent of the Toronto Asylum, Joseph Workman. Workman completely disagreed with Nelson. He responded with his statement of the principles upon which an asylum for criminal lunatics should be based.[61]

No lunatic asylum, whether intended for the lodgment of those called criminal, or any other class of the insane, should be regarded, or considered as a "penal institution." Insanity has never been cured, or benefited, by punitional measures. The primary object of all institutions for the insane is the restoration of the afflicted inmates to reason, or failing this, the attainment of the greatest possible amelioration of their unhappy condition: and at the present day, no second opinion exists among the members of the faculty of Psychology as to the character of the remedial agencies required for the desired object.[62]

Describing Nelson's punitive principles as "evils" of a "by-gone" era of pre-asylum patient treatment, Workman urged the government to continue with the architectural design of Rockwood as originally proposed. In so doing, he assured the provincial secretary, Canada would be following in the "foot-marks of our great and good mother land [England]" by building a "noble monument of national benevolence."[63]

This debate over the architecture of the new Rockwood asylum was finally resolved in favour of the opinions of Superintendent Workman, and the original plans were carried out. But an analysis of the debate itself underscores the inconsistency among the professional perspectives on the subject of criminal insanity. In

1855 Inspector Nelson had been a strong proponent of the medical treatment of criminal insanity as a distinct psychiatric entity. Yet only a few years later, he had come to favour the penal aspects of institutional management of the criminally insane. Conversely, Superintendent Workman, who was originally adamant that the criminally insane would corrupt the good management of his asylum for the "ordinary" insane, now appeared to endorse curative principles that applied equally to both classes of insane patients.

The shifting perspectives of influential professionals on the nature of criminal insanity and the best form for its institutional treatment coincided with developments at the community level that seriously affected the composition of the patient population at Rockwood. When the criminal lunatic asylum was first established in 1855, asylum inspectors had been concerned about the general lack of accommodation available for the non-criminal insane. "The Beauport Asylum in Canada East," they reported, "[was] thronged to excess, whilst that at Toronto has been compelled to reject numerous applications." The inspectors therefore advised that the new asylum at Rockwood should contain a ward for ordinary lunatics to help offset the overcrowded state of the other institutions.[64] By the time the new Rockwood asylum was nearing completion a decade later in 1868, the crisis in accommodation for the non-criminal insane had become even more acute.

The municipalities in the eastern counties of Upper Canada partially solved this crisis of space by manipulating the laws governing admission to Rockwood. When the asylum first opened, the provincial secretary made the legal differentiation between the criminal insane and the ordinary insane clear to Superintendent Litchfield. A lunatic whose legal status fell under the 4th section of Act 14th and 15th Vict. Ch. 83, would, upon proper notification to His Excellency, be removed from a local jail to the criminal lunatic asylum. On the other hand, lunatics "committed to jail as being furiously mad, and endangering the persons and properties of themselves or others under the 5th section of the same act, and [who] have not been charged with or convicted of any crime … cannot be removed to the [criminal lunatic asylum,] as they do not come within the character of criminal lunatics.[65]

According to Litchfield, the original intent of the law for admission to the criminal lunatic asylum was undermined by the public through the criminalization of ordinary cases of insanity. This criminalization was achieved by "tacking" onto an ordinary lunatic an official charge of assault, or being dangerous to the public. In this way, the ordinary lunatic was labelled an insane offender and "committed to gaol as the preliminary step to a transfer to the Criminal Lunatic Asylum." Litchfield argued that this legal manipulation helped to relieve problems of accommodation for the insane of the province, and enabled municipalities close to Rockwood to avoid spending large sums of money transporting insane persons to the more distant Toronto Provincial Asylum. Finally, this rediagnosis of the ordinary insane alllowed their families in the near vicinity of Rockwood to keep "their relatives as near to them, and in an asylum as convenient of access for them" as possible.[66]

By 1868 when the new Rockwood Criminal Lunatic Asylum was finally ready to receive all the patients from the temporary asylums, this practice of committing the ordinary insane as criminal lunatics through "evasion of the law" had considerably altered the balance of Litchfield's patient population.[67] Patients who had actually committed a criminal offence and were thus considered criminally insane had become a small minority within a population of the ordinary insane. Accordingly, the new asylum, originally conceived as an institution for the treatment of the criminally insane, took on the role of a general asylum to serve the adjacent counties of Upper Canada.

In their efforts to deal with their own pressing concerns, the families of the insane, along with local municipal officials and other community members, adopted a strategy that substantially altered the institutional structure originally created to deal with the medico-therapeutic crisis of criminal insanity in mid-century Canada. Their successful transformation of the Rockwood Criminal Lunatic Asylum into an institution catering largely to the ordinary insane contributed to the erosion of the identity of the criminally insane as a specific deviant group requiring a particular form of medical institutional treatment. As superintendent of the medical experiment in institutional treatment of the criminally insane, Litchfield's reached conclusions about the similarities between criminal and ordinary forms of insanity that further eroded the medical and therapeutic distinctiveness of this group.

As the complex historical circumstances that had originally led to the medical definition of criminal insanity changed, criminal lunatics in Canada were again left in an ambiguous and ultimately more vulnerable position. Litchfield's decision to have criminal lunatic patients treated within the new Rockwood Asylum "in association with the ordinary insane" was quickly and forcefully contested after his death in 1868. Just one year after the transfer of all remaining criminal lunatics to the new asylum, Litchfield's successor, Superintendent Dickson, aggressively campaigned for the removal of "the criminal class of lunatics" from the Rockwood Asylum. Unlike Litchfield, Dickson saw "the criminal [as] a man of low, brutal instinct," adding that "this trait of his character ... always show[ed] itself whether he [was] sane or insane." He further argued that when the criminal lunatic was "placed in an Asylum among respectable [that is to say non-criminal] patients, instead of being influenced by any efforts that may be employed with the view of working some reformation of his character and conduct, he only seeks to pollute others ..." Dickson's view was that criminal lunatics "should never be permitted to go beyond the walls of the Penitentiary."[68] His persistence finally prompted an amendment of the *Penitentiary Act* in 1877, which paved the way for the transfer of Rockwood Asylum's criminal lunatics back to the Kingston Penitentiary.[69]

At the penitentiary, criminal lunatics were dealt with strictly as convicts; all pretense of medical diagnosis, treatment or care completely disappeared. The extent to which the prevailing outlook on criminal insanity had altered is evident in the observations of visiting English alienist Daniel Hack Tuke, who inspected the criminally insane at Kingston in 1884.

The patients are treated with almost as much rigour as convicts, though not dressed in prison garb ... In the basement are "dungeons," to which patients when they are refractory are consigned as a punishment, although the cells above are in all conscience sufficiently prison-like. The floors of the cells are of stone, and would be felt to be a punishment by any patient in the asylums of Ontario ... Two men in the cells had once been patients in the asylum. One, with whom we conversed at the iron gate of this dungeon, laboured under a distinct delusion of there being a conspiracy against him. It was certainly not very likely to be dispelled by the dismal stone-floor dungeon in which he was immured, without a seat, unless he chose to use the bucket intended for other purposes, which was the only piece of furniture in the room.[70]

In Tuke's view, this treatment of criminal lunatics was simply "wrong": "Either they are or are not lunatics," he wrote. "If they are, they ought to be differently cared for."[71] In the Kingston Penitentiary, the perception and treatment of the criminally insane as mere criminals persisted for thirty years after Tuke's visit. Finally, in 1914, a Royal Commission on Penitentiaries issued a scathing report on the condition of the criminal lunatics, after which the insane were permanently removed from the penitentiary.[72]

The emergence and subsequent disappearance of criminal insanity as an officially recognized psychiatric disorder in the nineteenth century offers a revealing case study in developing responses to insanity. As one aspect of a general crisis in Canada's first penitentiary at mid-century, criminal insanity took on the proportions of a major problem. But it had no easy solution. Criminal lunatics fit awkwardly into the limited range of institutional settings available in Ontario and Quebec.

In the course of the debate among medical and political officials over the appropriate means of dealing with this particular combination of crime and mental alienation, criminal insanity was temporarily classified as a specialized psychiatric disorder in need of a separate medical institution. This temporary consensus led to the establishment of the Rockwood Criminal Lunatic Asylum for the treatment of the criminally insane. However, for a variety of reasons, this tenuous psychiatric construct was short-lived and the institutionalized treatment of the criminally insane was soon abandoned.

Ironically, one of the principal causes of the declassification of criminal insanity as a psychiatric disorder in Canada was the demand by communities surrounding Rockwood for asylum provision for their non-criminal insane. The community was able to circumvent the laws governing the admission of criminal lunatics to Rockwood, thereby redefining the asylum that was originally intended for the treatment of a specialized form of insanity as an asylum primarily for the management of patients with no actual criminal histories. In this case, the community's needs and perceptions about the use of the asylum had a profound, if indirect, influence on the configuration of state and psychiatric policy towards the criminally insane. The brief episode of the psychiatric conceptualization of criminal insanity in nineteenth-century Canada also exemplifies the uneven development of the asylum as the institutional expression of state and psychiatric power.

Re-evaluating the Asylum,
the State, and the Management
of Insanity

In Quebec and Ontario the state played a major role in the social history of the asylum. Lunatic asylums in both provinces gradually became part of a bureaucratized institutional network presided over by the Inspectorate of Prisons, Asylums and Public Charities in 1859, and by separate state inspectorates for each province after Confederation. State involvement in institutions for the management and treatment of the insane was an aspect of a larger project of developing statehood in mid-nineteenth-century Canada encompassing educational and penal reform along with efforts to police and regulate other aspects of social life.[1]

The historical influence of the state in nineteenth-century Canadian educational development has been thoroughly explored by sociologist Bruce Curtis[2]. In Curtis's view, "systematic efforts were undertaken by the imperial government and the colonial Parliament to educate 'the people' in the ideological, moral and behavioral requisites of the new forms of governance" which accompanied the "extension of capitalist relations of production" and the consolidation of "liberal political democracy" at mid-century.[3] Central to this process was the establishment of an inspectorate to monitor and regulate, at the local level, the policies generated by the central state. Borrowing from Foucault, Curtis argues that government inspectors of all kinds facilitated the development of "panoptic" modes of state power.[4]

In some respects, Curtis's understanding of education and state formation appears relevant to a study of the development of the state lunatic asylum. Several historians have pointed out the ways in which the concept of the Victorian lunatic asylum embodied the ideals of bourgeois society. With a tremendous emphasis on order and control in its design and management, the asylum was designed to make irrational minds rational again, imbued with the values and habits of those who endorsed and controlled the asylum itself: middle-class philanthropists, asylum advocates, medical superintendents, and various state officials.[5] Through the practice of the doctrine of moral therapy, the insane would be cured and released from the asylum as productive members of society.[6] These institutions were to be controlled and supervised by an inspectorate that served as a channel of communication between those responsible for the daily affairs of the asylum and the officials of the state. The space in which the work of healing disordered minds took place was to be well regulated and directed by the state inspectorate as its expertise in the study and cure of insanity grew.

Moreover, there was a congruency between the objectives of the state asylum and those of an emerging psychiatric profession struggling for power and status in the medical field. The participation of medical superintendents in the process of state asylum development helped ensure an emphasis on the presumed objectivity of science and medicine in the reordering of disordered minds. The weight placed on the role of science and medicine in the cure of insanity would help to further legitimize the state's involvement in the institutional treatment and management of the insane as a rational and empirical enterprise.[7]

While these were the ideological tenets of the nineteenth-century state lunatic asylum, they only partially reflected the reality of state involvement in the care and management of the insane in Quebec and Ontario. The relationship between the state and insanity was quite different in each province. In Quebec, a peculiar arrangement developed whereby most of the state's efforts at regulation and control were effectively thwarted by a proprietary asylum system which, ironically, the state had helped to initiate. The Beauport Asylum's proprietors' successful resistance to state regulation gave them a virtual monopoly in the institutional management of insanity in Quebec from 1845 to 1873. This monopoly set the pattern for the relationship between the state and insanity throughout in the century. The prominent role of the Catholic Church in the sphere of charity work further contributed to the particular nature of state involvement in the treatment and management of the insane in that province. Although the farming-out system that developed in Quebec successfully resisted state interference and control for much of the nineteenth century, close organizational links were established between the state and the institutions that contracted for the care of pauper patients. More-over, the Beauport proprietors had a similar vision of the social and therapeutic purpose of the lunatic asylum as their non-pro-prietary alienist colleagues in Ontario and elsewhere. Thus, in important respects, their institution resembled those established through more direct state intervention in Ontario. But the propri-etary nature of the asylum movement in Quebec, along with the powerful influence of the Catholic Church later in the century, created a unique relationship between the state and insanity in Quebec.

In Ontario, a more conventional form of state-driven asylum management and treatment emerged. The first provisional asylum for the insane and the network of permanent asylums which fol-lowed were state-run, and developed into a relatively sophisticat-ed system of government-inspected institutions. Yet this process of state development in the sphere of institutionalized care of the insane was fraught with difficulties. Conflicts between asylum inspectors and superintendents demonstrated disagreement over the distribution of state power and differences in opinion as to the role of the asylum as a state institution. Community members also frequently voiced their opinions on the proper purpose of the lunatic asylum in Ontario – opinions that often differed from those of both the state and the medical superintendents. Because the construction and subsequent maintenance of lunatic asylums was largely funded by public monies in the form of a county asy-lum tax, Ontario communities were particularly sensitive to the government's involvement in the management and care of the insane. Moreover, the effective operation of a state institution for the insane in ways envisioned by asylum promoters and state offi-cials was delayed for decades in Ontario because of financial con-straints. Such deferment of intentions seriously undermined the state's regulation and control of insanity for much of the nine-teenth century.

In neither province did the asylum emerge out of a socio-therapeutic vacuum. A range of local practices in the treatment and management of insanity had preceded lunatic asylums and continued to
exist well after their introduction. These local, non-asylum socio-
medical practices are aspects of the history of insanity that deserve
more attention. Their existence and their perpetuation had an
important influence on the shaping of the lunatic asylum. An examination of the relationship between asylum medicine and patient
care in non-asylum contexts reveals as much about alienists' views
on insanity as it does about community-level perceptions of, and
responses to, those considered insane.

Individual families and community members further shaped the
character of asylum development in Ontario and Quebec as they
made their decisions to commit those they considered insane to
the new institutions. An analysis of the motives for asylum committal at the local level reveals a great disparity between state,
alienist, and community perceptions of the asylum. Individual
families and neighbours of the insane made strategic use of the
institution in ways that were inconsistent with the principles of
asylum medicine as expressed by medical superintendents. Social
and economic stresses in the household were more important than
medical considerations for most families who sought the admission of their relatives or acquaintances to the asylums of Ontario
and Quebec. And, when medicine did come to bear on decisions
for committal in the form of treatment by local doctors, it was
usually in a context decidedly in conflict with the medical philosophy of the insane asylum. These findings point toward the need
to reassess previous accounts of the asylum in nineteenth-century
society.

One of the major contributions of the first round of revisionist writing was its focus on the important role of the state in asylum development and in the regulation of madness. As the field of asylum
studies produces an ever richer picture of the manifold aspects of
asylum life (both inside and outside of the institution) this contribution ought not be forgotten. However, it is clear from the historically detailed and topically varied accounts of more recent studies
that neither a linear nor a "top-down" approach to the state's activities sufficiently explains the complex historical consequences of the
state's role in asylum building.

Andrew Scull has argued that the socioeconomic dislocations of capitalist development in England severely compromised the caring capacity of the family at the same time that the bourgeoisie established the state asylum for the containment of one of society's unproductive and increasingly visible groups.[8] In Gerald Grob's view, the good intentions of early state asylum advocates in the United States foundered on the major social and economic shifts in nineteenth-century American society.[9] Closer to home, Rainer Baehre has argued that Upper Canadian reform-minded politicians of varying political stripes viewed the state lunatic asylum as one of several innovations in the creation of a "new moral-legal world" or "common interest." To Baehre, the asylum was a manifestation of a cultural revolution in moral sentiment and an administrative revolution in rational government.[10]

Despite the range of views on state formation that these studies represent, what is missing in all of them is a close consideration of how the tensions and conflicts between psychiatric, state, and community interests shaped the state's response to insanity. An analysis of asylum development in Ontario and Quebec suggests that the actual process and impact of state development in the management of insanity was more complicated and uneven than has been previously suggested. The state asylum (like other state institutions such as the school, penitentiary, and reformatory) was recast in the nineteenth century by powerful middle and upper class groups who shared a broad set of concerns about reform and social control.[11] Furthermore, through the development of the asylum, the state did become a much more intrusive and powerful force in the management, definition, and treatment of insanity. But, as J.I. Little has recently argued, "to examine state formation only from the perspective of the government and its legislation is ... to leave oneself open to fundamental misunderstanding not only of the dynamics involved but of the impact institutional reform made on social and economic development ..."[12]

Bruce Curtis does give room for analysis of the relationship between local conflict and state formation. But he argues that "once set in motion, the administrative organization of public education produced its own developmental logic, in which local opposition contributed to the growth of administrative structure." In Curtis' view, "local opposition to central policy initiatives tended to extend and solidify administrative structures." Community response and opposition were contained and muted within the new educational state created at mid-century.[13]

As with education, the rise of the state lunatic asylum made it impossible for decisions at the local level to be separated from the decisions of those who held greater authority at the asylum and state levels in Quebec. The strategies of families in the process of asylum committal were vulnerable to the decisions of those in positions of greater power at the asylum and within the state apparatus. The mere act of petitioning activated a complex power hierarchy in which the average petitioner had to tread deferentially to achieve success. A close study of petitions for committal brings into sharp relief the uneven playing field upon which the competing outlooks of local petitioners and state and asylum officials played themselves out. And, once a person was committed, the power of the family and of the community over the management and care of the insane patient could be drastically reduced. In other words, the power and influence of each group that affected the course of state asylum building were not equal.

Nevertheless, the social history of insanity and asylum development in Quebec and Ontario demonstrates that no all-encompassing "psychiatric state" was established in the same way that Curtis has argued was the case for education. Disparities in power notwithstanding, the state lunatic asylum was the product of complex, conflicting relationships between state, psychiatric and community forces. The conflicts emanating from these relationships were never successfully contained by the state, and while an attendant set of values and understandings about insanity was stamped, it was by no means sealed by the interests of the state. Reformers and asylum promoters did manage to establish a state system of lunatic asylums, but in neither province did they do so just as they pleased.

Notes

ABBREVIATIONS

NA	National Archives of Canada
RG5 C1	Correspondence of the Provincial Secretary, Ontario
RG4 C1	Correspondence of the Provincial Secretary, Quebec
AO	Archives of Ontario
JLAUC	Journals of the Legislative Assembly of Upper Canada
JLHLC	Journals of the Legislative House of Lower Canada

INTRODUCTION

1 Sophie Bernier's story is drawn from the following source: *National Archives of Canada* (hereafter NA), RG4 C1, file 2294.

2 For the meliorist account see for example Gregory Zilboorg, *A History of Medical Psychology*, and Alexander and Selesnick, *The History of Psychiatry*. For the meliorist account in Canada see Burgess, "A Historical Sketch of Our Canadian Institutions for the Insane."

3 Foucault, *Folie et déraison*. The first publication in English of Foucault's work was *Madness and Civilization*. As Scull notes, the English translation was missing about 40 per cent of the content of the original French version, "as well as the bulk of the footnotes and references," a fact which helped fuel the tremendous intellectual controversy surrounding the book. Scull, "Reflections on the Historical Sociology of Psychiatry," 15.

174 Notes to pages 7–11

4 Among historians, much of the criticism of Foucault's sweeping interpretation has focused on problems of historical accuracy. See Middlefort, "Madness and Civilization"; Stone, *The Past and the Present Revisited*; Goldstein, "'The Lively Sensibility of the Frenchman'," 3–26; Porter, "Foucault's Great Confinement," 47–54.

5 Rothman, *The Discovery of the Asylum*; Scull, *Museums of Madness*. Other influential revisionist writings encompassing the grand sweep of geography, history, and theory include Doerner, *Madmen and the Bourgeoisie*; and Castel, *The Regulation of Madness*.

6 Scull situates himself in relation to Foucault's work in, "Reflections on the Historical Sociology of Psychiatry," 14–20; Scull, "Michel Foucault's History of Madness," 57–67; and Scull, "A Failure to Communicate?," 150–163. Rothman offers a brief critique of Foucault in Rothman, *Discovery of the Asylum*, xvii–xviii.

7 Perkin, *The Origins of Modern English Society*, 49, quoted in Scull, *The Most Solitary of Afflictions*, 30.

8 Grob, *The State and the Mentally Ill*; Grob, *Mental Institutions in America*

9 Both Grob and Scull have remained influential figures in the field. While their perspectives have become more nuanced and contextualized, both historians have held relatively fast to their respective positions on the development of the asylum. See Grob, *Mental Illness and American Society*; Grob, *From Asylum to Community*; Grob, *The Mad Among Us*; Scull, *Social Order/Mental Disorder*; Scull, *The Most Solitary of Afflictions*. Grob and Scull have frequently been each other's most vociferous critic, bringing into stark relief the differences in their perspectives. See for example Grob, "Marxian Analysis and Mental Illness." Scull returns the favour in Scull, "Mental Health Policy in Modern America." Of historiographical note is also Rothman's long introduction to the 1990 re-edition of his earlier classic. Rothman, *Discovery of the Asylum*, xiii–xliv.

10 Some academics continued this debate into the 1980s and 1990s.

11 Included in this outpouring of recent literature is: Finnane, *Insanity and the Insane in Post-Famine Ireland*; Tomes, *A Generous Confidence*; Digby, *Madness, Morality and Medicine*; Showalter, *The Female Malady*; Shortt, *Victorian Lunacy*; Dwyer, *Homes for the Mad*; Porter, *Mind-Forg'd Manacles*; Warsh, *Moments of Unreason*; Ripa, *Women and Madness*; Peter McCandless, *Moonlight, Magnolias and Madness*.

12 The phrase is borrowed from Thompson, *The Making of the English Working Class*, 12.

13 Brown, "Dance of the Dialectic?," 28

14 Ibid., 26

15 Peter Keating, *La science du mal*, 30

16 "Above all," states Shorter, "I have tried to rescue the history of psychiatry from the sectarians who have made the subject a sandbox for their ideologies. To an extent unimaginable for other areas of the history of medicine, zealot researchers have seized the history of psychiatry to illustrate how their pet bugaboos – be they capitalism, patriarchy, or psychiatry itself – have converted protest into illness, locking into asylum those who otherwise would be challenging the established order." Shorter, *A History of Psychiatry*, viii

17 Shorter, *A History of Psychiatry*, vii

18 Wright, "Getting Out of the Asylum"

19 Ibid., 139. Wright points to the merger of asylum and family history as one way in which a reconceptualization of the history of insanity could proceed.

20 This focus on the family and the community context has led to a questioning of the the centrality of the asylum itself in nineteenth-century histories of insanity. See for example Bartlett and Wright eds., *Outside the Walls of the Asylum*. For the American context see Moran, "Asylum in the Community."

21 One aspect of the history of the asylum that is largely absent in this book is that of patient experience. This subject has been the focus of the important work of Geoffrey Reaume. See Reaume *999 Queen Street West*.

CHAPTER ONE

1 Part of the grant for the insane was allocated for the boarding out of a small number of lunatics to families in the country. In 1823, for example, five of twenty insane persons in Quebec were boarded out by the state to families in the province. See Report of a Committee on Insane Persons and Foundlings, *Journals of the Legislative House of Lower Canada* (hereafter JLHLC), vol. 33, 1824–25.

2 Much of this criticism focused on how to expand and improve provision at the general hospitals. See for example, "Report of a Committee on the Petition of the Commissioners for Insane Persons and Foundlings," *JLHLC*, 31 January 1818.

3 W. Hackett, "Mémoire au Gouverneur Sherbrooke," 27 October 1816 in "Rapport du Comité Spécial nommé pour s'enquérIr et faire rapport sur les établissements de cette province, pour la réception et la guérisson des Personnes dérangées dans leur esprit," *Journals of the Legislative Council* (hereafter JLC), 1824, (appendix 1).

4 NA, RG4 B65, Grand Jury Presentment, July 1844, file 3064

5 See for example "Rapport du Comité spécial" *Journaux de L'Assemblée Législative*, 1824, appendix 1 (Bas Canada). It is important to point out

that a serious historiographical debate between Cellard and Keating exists over the *système des loges* and their perceived therapeutic efficacy. In *La science du mal*, Keating argues that the practice of moral therapy actually began to take root in the general hospitals of Lower Canada. Focusing on the six "cellules morales" under the medical guidance of A.F. Holmes at the Hôpital Général de Québec, Keating argues that moral treatment of the insane had already developed in a pre-asylum context. From his reading of the evidence, Keating concluded that moral treatment was not singularly the ideological justification or theoretical expression of the insane asylum itself. See Keating, *La science du mal*, 53. Cellard strongly objects to this reading of the *système des loges*. For Cellard's side of the story see *Histoire de la folie au Québec*, 169–179.

6   "Message from the Lieutenant Governor relating to the Insane and Lunatics of the Province, and recommending the building of a Lunatic Asylum," 1 March 1825, *JLHLC*.

7   Ibid.

8   See for example, NA, RG4 C1, file 1489, Grand Jury Presentment, July 1843.

9   Keating, *La science du mal*, 47

10   See NA, RG4 C1, file 2056, Petition of the Inhabitants of Montreal Calling for the Establishment of a Lunatic Asylum, 1842.

11   Ibid.

12   See Doratt, "Observations on the Custody of the Insane and the Expediency of a Public Lunatic Asylum," Appendix 3, *Lord Durham's Report on the Affairs of British North America.*

13   These figures were conservative in comparison to those boasted by several prominent alienists of the day.

14   Doratt, "Observations"

15   As Rothman puts it, "The first postulate of the asylum program was the prompt removal of the insane from the community. As soon as the first symptom of the disease appeared, the patient had to enter a mental hospital. Medical superintendents unanimously and without exception asserted that treatment within the family was doomed to fail." Rothman, *Discovery of the Asylum*, 137

16   Cellard further points out that the arrival during the 1830s of large numbers of immigrants from Britain, many in desperate social and economic straits, strengthened the perception among colonial and imperial officials that state institutions were needed in the colony to effect social order. Finally, argues Cellard, the growing agricultural crisis in Lower Canada, in precipitating the urbanization of many French Canadians and in undermining the family's ability to cope with dependent family members, contributed to the perceived need for state management of the insane. Cellard, *Histoire de la folie*, Chap. 3, passim

17 Ibid., 204.
18 See Allan Greer, "The Birth of the Police in Canada," and Brian Young, "Positive Law, Positive State."
19 See for example, NA RG4 C1, "Petition of the Inhabitants of Montreal Calling for the Establishment of a Lunatic Asylum," 1842. A similar petition appears in the same record group dated December 1844. Regular appeals for the establishment of a lunatic asylum for the district of Montreal were voiced by the editors of the *Canada Medical Journal*, published out of Montreal. See for example, *Canada Medical Journal*, July 1865, 45–47; *Ibid.*, April 1865, 491–2. See also, RG4 C1, file 1489, Grand Jury Presentment, July 1843; and file 712, Grand Jury Presentment, 1843. The Chairman and Secretary of the temporary asylum at Montreal, both former members of the Committee for the Establishment of a Permanent Lunatic Asylum appointed by Colbourne, also criticized the state of provision at the Montreal Jail and lobbied for the establishment of a permanent asylum. See NA, RG4 C1, file 1731, John Boston and J. Trestler to the Governor General, August 23 1843.
20 NA, RG4 C1, file 2204, "Memorial of Dorothea Dix to the Provincial Parliament of Canada East and West;" Dix to Charles Metcalfe, Governor in Chief of the United Provinces, 12 October 1843.
21 NA, RG4 C1, file 3064, "Governor General's Minutes on the Subject of Establishing a Lunatic Asylum in Lower Canada," 19 August 1844.
22 Ibid.
23 NA, RG4 C1, file 3064, Report of a Committee of the Executive Council … on the Several Papers Relating to the Establishment of Lunatic Asylums in Lower Canada, 19 September 1844
24 Ibid.
25 NA, RG4 C1, file 3064, Drs Badgely and Sutherland to Provincial Secretary, 20 November 1844
26 NA, RG4 C1, file 2888, Petition of Henry Mount to the Provincial Secretary, 2 September 1844; file 3064, Henry Mount to Provincial Secretary, 23 November 1844. It is unclear how much money per patient Mount expected to be paid in this arrangement.
27 NA, RG4 C1, file 3064, James Douglas to Provincial Secretary, 18 November 1844. During these negotiations, proposals for the establishment of a permanent lunatic asylum were sent to the government from other sources. See for example the petition of the inhabitants of Trois Rivières "que la ville de Trois Rivières soit choisie pour y ériger un Hôpital pour les insensés." NA, RG4 C1, file 3772
28 NA, RG4 C1, "Report of a Committee of the Executive Council," 28 April 1845; RG4 C1, files 787–90, Provincial Secretary to Trestler, 1 May 1845; Provincial Secretary to Dr. Mount, 1 May 1845; Provincial Secretary to Drs. Badgely and Sutherland, 1 May 1845

29   NA, RG4 C1, Provincial Secretary to Drs. Douglas, Morrin and Frémont,
      1 May 1845

30   NA, RG4 C1, file 1517, James Douglas to Provincial Secretary, 14 May
      1845; James Douglas to Provincial Secretary, 15 June 1845; Report of a
      Committee of the Executive Council, 18 June 1845; RG4 C1, file 1523,
      Provincial Secretary to Douglas, Frémont and Morrin, no date

31   NA, RG4 C1, Dr Trestler to Provincial Secretary, 23 June 1845

32   NA, RG4 C1, file 2984, Report of a Committee of the Executive Council,
      30 June 1845; Badgely and Sutherland to Provincial Secretary, 11 July
      1845; RG4 C1, Provincial Secretary to F. Badgely and D. Sutherland, 5
      July 1845

33   Trestler, the secretary of the temporary asylum at Montreal, who was on
      the original committee struck by Colbourne that purchased the St
      Antoine site for a state asylum in 1839, was by now very frustrated:
      "When I think that in Lower Canada, when there are about 1200 *non
      compos mentis* – you hardly find any convenient place to receive some
      of them – it makes one feel mal à ton aise. There ought to be at least
      one asylum in Montreal, Three Rivers and Quebec, and they would
      shortly be filled up." NA, RG4 C1, file 2224, Trestler to John Boston, 24
      July 1845; see also Dr. Dan Arnoldi physician to the Montreal Gaol to
      Sheriff Coffin, 11 July 1845; Thomas McGuinn, Gaoler to Boston and
      Coffin, 23 July 1845.

34   NA, RG4 C1, file 1855, Report of a Committee of the Executive Council,
      11 August 1845

35   See for example NA, RG4 C1, file 4101, "Report on Cases of Lunatics
      Confined in Montreal Gaol," 23 December 1847; Thomas McGinn to
      Dan Arnoldi, 2 December 1847.

36   NA, RG4 C1, file 2191, "Jean Baptiste Curtius Trestler, MD Prays for the
      Establishment of a Lunatic Asylum in Montreal," 17 July 1848. Trestler's
      petition was endorsed by the Grand Mgr L'Evêque of Montreal.

37   NA, RG4 C1, Report of the Executive Committee, no date, filed with 135
      of 1846

38   NA, RG4 C1, file 2567, Memorandum to the Provincial Secretary from
      the Beauport Proprietors, 25 August 1848

39   Ibid.

40   NA, RG4 C1, file 2567, Memorandum of the Provincial Secretary, 12 Sep-
      tember 1848

41   NA, RG4 C1, file 2567, James Douglas to Provincial Secretary, 26 Septem-
      ber 1848; Report of the Executive Committee, 4 October 1848. In the
      renewed contract, the asylum proprietors promised to have the proposed
      new building completed within one year of the renewal date of the con-
      tract, "in default" of which they consented "that the present contract
      shall terminate at the expiration of five years." This undertaking proba-

bly helped convince the state of the proprietors' seriousness in regard to their proposed improvements of the physical plant of the asylum and the classification of patients according to contemporary medical standards.

42 See for example NA, RG4 C1, file 252, Provincial Secretary's response to Dr Henry Mount's proposal to establish an asylum at Montreal, 7 February 1852.

43 NA, RG4 C1, file 3118, Drs. Douglas, Frémont and Morrin to Provincial Secretary, 7 November 1848

44 For a full description of the new asylum and grounds see NA, RG4 C1, file 866, Annual Report of the Commissioners of the Beauport Lunatic Asylum, 27 April 1850.

45 NA, RG4 C1, file 1908, Memorandum of the Proprietors and Managers of the Quebec Lunatic Asylum, 24 November 1853; James Douglas to Provincial Secretary, 20 January 1854

46 NA, RG4 C1, file 1908, Memorandum of the Provincial Secretary, 20 February 1854. In order to fulfill the obligations of the new contract, the provincial secretary recommended that the annual state allocation of funds be increased from £7,500 to £9,100. The Provincial Secretary noted that £7,500 was the annual legislative allotment for Upper Canada for the care of the insane, and that the Upper Province was also likely to increase its allocation for this purpose to £9,100.

47 NA, RG4 C1, file 2880, Morrin, Frémont and Douglas to Provincial Secretary, 3 December 1856; Provincial Secretary to Morrin, Frémont and Douglas, 17 December 1856; Beauport Proprietors to Provincial Secretary, 25 December 1856; Provincial Secretary to Beauport Proprietors, 7 April 1857; Beauport Proprietors to Provincial Secretary, 4 April 1857; RG4 B65, file 690, Provincial Secretary to Charles Frémont, 20 April 1857

48 See NA, RG4 B65, file 193, Provincial Secretary's Memorandum on the Grant to the Beauport Lunatic Asylum, 4 February 1857; Copy of Report of a Committee of the Executive Council ... Approved by the Governor General 9 February 1857; A. Lemoine, Secretary to the Commissioners of the Beauport Lunatic Asylum to Provincial Secretary, 9 February 1857; E. Parent to A. Lemoine, 20 February 1857; Douglas, Morrin and Frémont to Provincial Secretary, 27 February 1857; Lemoine to Provincial Secretary, 12 October 1858; Morrin and Frémont to Lemoine, 6 April 1859

49 NA, RG4 C1, file 1572, Parent to Dr. Frémont, 31 May 1862

50 NA, RG4 C1, Solicitor General to Prison Inspectors, 17 June 1864; Secretary of the Board of Inspectors to Solicitor General, 26 June 1864

51 Ibid.

52 Ironically, in the face of these criticisms, requests by the government for the Beauport proprietors to increase their accommodation of the insane

who were confined in the local jails went on unabated. On 1 July 1863, 25 insane prisoners were transferred from the Montreal Jail alone to the Beauport Lunatic Asylum.

53 NA, RG4 C1, file 1772, Landry and Douglas to Provincial Secretary, 11 July 1864

54 NA, RG4 C1, file 2675, Douglas and Landry to Provincial Secretary, 5 December 1864

55 NA, RG4 C1, file 1772, Douglas and Landry to Provincial Secretary, December 29 1864

56 NA, RG4 C1, file 2675, Douglas to Provincial Secretary, 15 April 1865

57 In addition to the objections articulated by the proprietors to certain key terms proposed by the government, Douglas and Landry had their own demands. As previously mentioned, they wanted the ceiling clause in the new contract for government patients to be set at 750. Second, Douglas and Landry wanted a clause in the contract protecting them against a sudden rise in the price of goods and labour in the event of a war with the United States. Their third major demand was that a ten-year contract be struck in order that the money expended in asylum expansion could be recovered.

58 NA, RG4 C1, file 2675, Douglas to Provincial Secretary, 15 April 1865. Both signed under protest with the following note to the provincial secretary: "In conformity with our promise, we propose signing a new contract. We wish it however to be distinctly understood that we do so under protest, and with the intention of appealing to the council for the revision of its conditions, whenever the council shall reassemble. We intend applying for redress to those members especially who last summer pledged themselves to a renewal of the existing contract on condition of our affording additional accommodation for the insane of the province. We have fulfilled our part, and do not consider the so called contract now offered us, as a fulfilment of theirs. We sign, because forced to do so by the undue pressure and intimidation."

59 NA, RG4 C1, file 2675, Douglas to Provincial Secretary, 15 April 1865; see also McDougall to Douglas, 19 April 1865, where the provincial secretary attempts to allay Douglas's fears about government interference.

60 NA, RG4 C1, file 1, James Douglas Jr to Provincial Secretary, 30 December 1865; Report of the Executive Council, 6 January 1866; Assistant Provincial Secretary to Douglas, Landry and Roy, 9 January 1866

61 Interestingly, Roy's early complaints were mitigated by reports from Dr Taché, a member of the Board of Inspectors who was generally sympathetic to the proprietors of the Beauport Asylum. Taché noted that, although the visiting physician's concerns were valid in some respects, prior to Roy's appointment the proprietors had made considerable efforts to improve conditions in the attic wards. Taché's reports dimin-

ished the urgency of Roy's recommendations in the eyes of the state. NA, RG4 CI, file 2068, Report of Visiting Physician Dr Roy, 6 June 1865; Taché to Provincial Secretary, 6 June 1865; RG4 B65, file 1437, Report of Visiting Physician Dr Roy, 1 September 1865; Report of Visiting Physician Dr Roy, 3 October 1865

62 NA, RG4 CI, file 2392, "Copie de quelques remarques faites par le médecin visiteur sur l'Asile des Aliénés à Beauport," 6 October to 30 October 1865

63 NA, RG4 CI, file 2392, Provincial Secretary to Secretary to the Commissioners of the Beauport Lunatic Asylum, 8 February 1866; Provincial Secretary to Roy, 31 October 1865; Inspector Taché to Provincial Secretary, 21 December 1865; Roy to Assistant Provincial Secretary, 24 January 1866; Assistant Provincial Secretary to Roy, 10 February 1866

64 A brief description of events is given by James Douglas Jr in, *Journals and Reminiscences of James Douglas*, 217.

65 To get a sense of the battles between Dr A. Jackson and the asylum proprietors, see NA, RG4 CI, file 1809, Report of Visiting Physician Dr A. Jackson on the Beauport Lunatic Asylum to Provincial Secretary, 18 September 1866; Jackson Report to Provincial Secretary, 7 January 1867; Provincial Secretary to Secretary of the Commissioners of the Beauport Lunatic Asylum, 18 January 1867; Landry and Roy to Provincial Secretary, 28 January 1867; Jackson to N.F. Belham, 21 February 1867; Landry and Roy to Assistant Provincial Secretary, 17 March 1867.

66 Inhabitants of St Francis, Sherbrooke, La Prairie, Terrebonne, and Montreal all petitioned at various stages for state funds to build asylums. These petitions made it clear to the government that the Beauport Asylum (and, later on, the St Jean Asylum) was unable to adequately provide for the large numbers of insane in the province. Concern was raised that this inadequacy resulted in the detention of patients in the local jails of the community, which in turn deprived the insane of the "necessary medical attendance to mitigate or remove the ailments." There is no evidence that these community-based petitions were paid any heed by the government. See NA, RG4 CI, file 1221, Petition of the Inhabitants of St Francis, 31 March 1846; file 846, Petition of the Inhabitants of Sherbrooke, February 1856; file 1857, Petition of the Inhabitants of La Prairie, 8 July 1862; file 2124, On the Establishment of an Asylum at Terrebonne, 6 August 1862. Similar sentiments on the need for increased accommodation for the insane were expressed in several Grand Jury Presentments. See for example NA, RG4 CI, file 2521, Report of the Grand Jury, Montreal, 18 October 1852.

67 Private proposals raised some of the same concerns as the community petitions. But they were also decidedly more entrepreneurial in form. Dr Henry Mount, one of the first medical entrepreneurs to negotiate with

the state back in 1845, petitioned again in 1848, and in 1852, to "establish a lunatic asylum near the city of Montreal under the auspices of Government." See *NA*, RG4 C1, file 2601, Dr Mount to Provincial Secretary, 1848; file 252, Dr Henry Mount to Provincial Secretary, 29 January 1852; Provincial Secretary to Henry Mount, 7 February 1852; Mount to Provincial Secretary, 7 February 1852. See also the petition of Dr A.H. David, *NA*, RG4 C1, file 534, Dr A.H. David to Provincial Secretary, 1 March 1859; file 459, David to Provincial Secretary, 6 March 1859; Provincial Secretary to David, 7 March 1859; file 930, David to Provincial Secretary, 5 April 1862. See also the petition of Wakeham, proprietor of the small Belmont Retreat for the insane. *NA*, RG4 C1, file 2578, G. Wakeham to Provincial Secretary, 17 November 1864; Provincial Secretary to Wakeham, 17 November 1864; File 29, Secretary to Commissioners of the Beauport Asylum to Solicitor General, 7 January 1865; Secretary of the Commissioners of the Beauport Asylum to Provincial Secretary, 5 January 1865. Also interested in more proprietary arrangements for the management and care of the insane was a group of former officials connected with the Temporary Lunatic Asylum in Montreal during its six year existence from 1839-1845. Dr Jean Trestler, former commissioner of, and physician to, the temporary lunatic asylum, petitioned the government several times. Trestler had the advantage of the official endorsement of his plans from the Bishop of Montreal. See *NA*, RG4 C1, file 2191, Trestler to Provincial Secretary, 17 July 1848; file 1500, Trestler to Provincial Secretary, 16 July 1851; file 1885, Trestler to Provincial Secretary, 25 August 1852. Similar overtures to the state were made by Edward Worth, former superintendent of the Temporary Lunatic Asylum in Montreal. See, *NA*, RG4 C1, file 236, Edward Worth to Provincial Secretary, 25 January 1849; file 1885, Worth to Provincial Secretary 25 August 1852.

68 NA, RG4 C1, file 252, Provincial Secretary to Henry Mount

69 See for example the report of Dr Nelson on the possibility of using Nicolet College for a lunatic asylum. NA, RG4 C1, file 1697, Wolfred Nelson to Provincial Secretary, 17 August 1861. See also de Bleury's offer of his 416-acre property at St Vincent de Paul for use as an asylum, NA, RG4 C1, file 2185, 14 August 1862.

70 NA, RG4 C1, file 557, Memorandum of the Provincial Secretary, 28 March 1861; "Rapport conjoint de M.M. les Docteurs Workman et Taché sur l'état actuel des propriétés ... à St. Jean et sur leur adaptabilité [pour un] Asile d'Aliénés," 2 mai 1860

71 Report of Inspector Taché, *Quebec Sessional Papers*, no. 66, 1863

72 NA, RG4 B65, file 1838, Howard to Provincial Secretary, 23 November 1861; RG4 B65, file 2748, Inspector Taché to Provincial Secretary, 13 December 1861

73 NA, RG4 C1, file 1698, Howard to Provincial Secretary, 19 August 1861; RG4 C1, file 2434, Taché to Provincial Secretary, 15 September 1862

74 See for example NA, RG4 C1, file 2412.

75 NA, RG4 C1, file 2522, John Palmer Litchfield to Provincial Secretary, 10 October 1863; Litchfield to Provincial Secretary, 19 December 1863

76 "Report of the Board of Inspectors on the Beauport Lunatic Asylum," *Sessional Papers*, No. 6, 1866, 6

77 "Report of the Board of Inspectors of Prisons, Asylums, and Public Charities," 30 December 1885, *Quebec Sessional Papers*, no. 10

78 See Act 48 Vict., chap. 34. As Peter Keating points out, this act had been preceded by three orders-in-council in 1879, which aimed to strengthen the power of the state-appointed visiting physician in relation to the Beauport and St Jean de Dieu Asylums. Keating, *La science du mal*, 88–90

79 Information on the medical boards has been gleaned from various passages of the *Report of the Royal Commission on Lunatic Asylum of the Province of Quebec, 1888*. For an extended discussion of the 1885 law, see Keating, *La science du mal*, 95–102.

80 See *Report of the Royal Commission on Lunatic Asylums*, passim.

81 Ibid., 72–9.

82 In addition to examining Beauport and St Jean de Dieu Asylums, the Royal Commission also studied three small institutions: the Belmont Retreat, the St Benoît Joseph Asylum, and the St Ferdinand d'Halifax Asylum.

83 See *Royal Commission on Lunatic Asylums*, 60–79

84 Ibid., 48, 50

85 Ibid

86 Ibid., 81, 169

87 Ibid., 50–2, 174

88 Keating, *La science du mal*, 108–9

89 Goldstein, *Console and Classify*, 198

90 As Goldstein puts it, "the Idéologues had placed consolation among the moral means available to the physician ... and Pinel had placed consolation first among the 'ways of gentleness' available to the physician employing the moral treatment on the insane; but in matters of consolation, the medical man was the amateur and the cleric the expert and past master." Goldstein, *Console and Classify*, 204

91 Ibid., 361–70

CHAPTER TWO

1 Rosenberg, *The Care of Strangers*, 47

2 See *Statutes of Upper Canada*, 11 Geo. IV, c. 20, 1830; and 3 Wm IV., c. 45, 1833.

3 See for example NA, RG4 B65, loose documents, Toronto Sheriff to Provincial Secretary, 16 September 1840. See also Oliver, '*Terror to Evil-Doers*', 44–5.

4 For a detailed account of the lack of action for the institutionalization of the insane in an asylum see Brown, "*Living with God's Afflicted*", 43–92.

5 Statutes of Upper Canada, 2 Vict., c. 10, 1839.

6 The decision to locate the temporary asylum in Toronto had not been unopposed. There was in fact a fierce debate between the medical profession in Kingston and Toronto over which city would establish the state institution. See, for example, NA RG5 C1, file 1198, "The petition of the College of Physicians and Surgeons in Toronto against the Provincial Lunatic Asylum being established in Kingston," 9 June 1840.

7 Rees's application for the post along with pertinent information about his medical career leading up to his appointment can be found in NA, RG5 C1, file 257, Rees to Provincial Secretary, 24 January 1840; Memorial of William Rees, 23 January 1840.

8 The eight additions were: Surgeon W.R. Beaumont, William Cawthra, Esq., John Eastwood, Esq., Rev. H.J. Grassett, Rev. J.J. Hay, William Kelly, Esq., Martin J. O'Bierne, Esq. and Rev. John Roaf.

9 This summary of duties and responsibilities has been drawn from NA, RG5 C1, file 2883, Report of the Commissioners and Proposed Rules and Regulations, 17 February 1841. These rules and regulations were significantly revised in 1854 as Superintendent Joseph Workman's powerful influence in the permanent Toronto Lunatic Asylum emerged.

10 See Rothman's classic work *The Discovery of the Asylum*.

11 American alienist Thomas Kirkbride turned this aspect of the lunatic asylum into a specialty. See Tomes, *A Generous Confidence*, 129–88.

12 Brown, "Architecture as Therapy"

13 The financial troubles of the temporary asylum are documented in NA, RG5 C1, file 3376, Grand Jury Report on the State of the Jail Lunatic Asylum, 4 April 1842; RG5 C1, file 5095, Superintendent Rees to Provincial Secretary, 24 November 1842; RG5 C1, file 5965, Rees to Provincial Secretary, 26 June 1843; RG5 C1, file 16645, Commissioner Grasett to Provincial Secretary, 1847.

14 See NA, RG5 C1, file 10418, copy of Grand Jurors' Report, 19 April 1844.

15 These examples were taken from NA, RG5 C1, file 7898, Rees to Board of Commissioners, 6 May 1844.

16 NA, RG5 C1, file 7898, "Special Report on the Toronto Lunatic Asylum by a Committee of the Board of Commissioners," 1844. The report was written by Commissioners John Roaf, Henry Grassett, and William Beaumont.

17 NA, RG5 C1, file 10418, Rees to Provincial Secretary, 4 April 1845

18 NA, RG5 C1, file 10418, "Report of a Committee of the Commissioners of the Temporary Lunatic Asylum"

19 NA, RG5 C1, file 10418, Rees to Provincial Secretary, 24 June 1845. The quotation from Philippe Pinel: "Whatever may be the principles on which an asylum is conducted, whatever locality and different forms of government the physician by the nature of his studies, the extent of his knowledge and the strong interest which he has in the success of treatment must be so well informed as to be the natural Judge of every thing that passes in an hospital for the insane." The quotation from Etienne Esquirol: "The physician should be the vital principle of an insane asylum. It is by him that every thing is put in motion, called as he is to be the regulator of all thoughts, he directs all actions. Everything which interests the inmates of the establishment points to him as the centre of action. The physician should be invested with authority from which no person can escape."

20 NA, RG5 C1, file 11903, Meeting of the commissioners for superintending the Temporary Lunatic Asylum, 15 October 1845

21 NA, RG5 C1, file 19774, Commissioners' Report, 23 March 1848. The commissioners also recommended the dismissal of the steward and matron on similar grounds.

22 NA, RG5 C1, file 19776, Telfer to Provincial Secretary, 2 April 1848; Provincial Secretary to Telfer, 17 April 1848; RG4 C1, file 20131, John Ewart to Provincial Secretary, 3 May 1848; testimony of Telfer to Provincial Secretary, 2 May 1848; Provincial Secretary to Telfer, 27 May 1848. This testimony, of course, suggests a certain disunity among some of the commissioners of the board. Further investigation into the relations between commissioners might prove a productive avenue of research. However, the fact that most major decisions were agreed upon by a majority of the board is critical to this study. Moreover the membership of the board remained very consistent until the formation of the Board of Inspectors of Prisons, Asylum,s and Public Charities in 1858.

23 NA, RG5 C1, file 19776, Provincial Secretary to Telfer, 17 April 1848; RG5 C1, file 20131, Provincial Secretary to Telfer, 27 May 1848

24 NA, RG5 C1, file 19815, Rev. Commissioner John Roaf to Provincial Secretary, 28 May 1848. Though denied the position, Scott would later be chosen as the first superintendent of the permanent lunatic asylum in Toronto.

25 NA, RG5 C1, file 512, Superintendent Parks to Provincial Secretary, 13 September 1848

26 See Minutes of Acting Superintendent Rolph to the Board of Commissioners, 11 August 1848, reproduced in Park, *A Narrative of the Recent Difficulties*, 6–7.

27 Ibid., 14, Rolph to Park, 8 September 1848
28 Ibid., John Rolph to the Board of Commissioners, 20 August 1848; Meeting of the Board of Commissioners, 29 August 1848.
29 See NA, RG5 C1, file 512, Park to the Board of Commissioners, 15 September 1848; Special Meeting Called by Weekly Commissioner, 12 September 1848, reproduced in Park, *A Narrative of the Recent Difficulties*, 18.
30 NA, RG5 C1, file 512, Park to the Board of Commissioners, 15 September 1848
31 NA, RG5 C1, file 512, extract from a Report of the Executive Council, 14 October 1848
32 NA, RG5 C1, file 512, Commissioners to the Provincial Secretary, 6 November 1848; Executive Council to the Commissioners, 29 November 1848
33 Particularly heated debate is reported over attendant Craig, who, despite continual suspension on charges of violence to patients, drunkenness, and disorderly conduct towards the matron, was persistently reinstated by the commissioners. Detail on this conflict can be found in Park, *A Narrative of the the Recent Difficulties*, passim.
34 NA, RG5 C1, file 1015, extract of a Report of a Committee of the Executive Council, 20 December 1848
35 Park, *A Narrative of the Recent Difficulties*, 49–50
36 Ibid., 28, 30, and 44
37 Brown notes that Scott's appointment and the retention of the old commissioners were heavily criticized by Toronto's *Examiner* and *Globe* newspapers. See Brown, *Living with God's Afflicted*, 150–2.
38 The member of the opposition was W.H. Boulton, former chair of the Commissioners for the Erection of a Permanent Lunatic Asylum. The suggestion led to substantial argument among members of parliament. See Brown, *Living With God's Afflicted*, 154.
39 As Brown points out, any bylaws made by the board were to be "subject to final approval by the government." Ibid. 159
40 NA, RG5 C1, file 148, Rules and Regulations for the Provincial Lunatic Asylum at Toronto, passed 17 June 1854.
41 This inability to lay blame may have been convenient. It is presumable that Workman became familiar with the close relationship between some of the asylum employees and individual commissioners.
42 NA, RG5 C1, file 1243, Report of the Superintendent to the Board of Commissioners, 1854
43 Ibid.
44 Ibid.
45 See Rosenberg, *The Care of Strangers*, Part I, "A Traditional Institution, 1800–1850," passim.
46 On the more "legitimate" form of perquisites associated with the role of asylum attendent, see Moran, "Keepers of the Insane."

47 For evidence of the persistence of an attendant/patient subculture which militated against the well-ordered institution see Ibid.

48 See for example Workman's accusations that the commissioners, "under the influence of the Bursar," changed the rules and regulations to increase the power of the bursar, NA, RG5 C1, file 7, Workman to Board of Commissioners, 2 January 1856; Memorial of the Commissioners to the Provincial Secretary; see also the debate over Workman's controversial dismissal of the asylum porter, RG5 C1, file 360; see also RG5 C1, file 620, Superintendent's Report to Commissioners, 22 March 1856.

49 They would not be completed until 1867 because of difficulties in raising money for their construction. See NA, RG5 C1, file 16377, Report of Architect John G. Howard, 26 February 1847; RG5 C1, file 17735, extract from a Report of a Committee of the Executive Council, 21 August 1847; RG5 C1, file 75, Statement of Moneys and Debentures Received by the Commissioners for Erecting the Provincial Lunatic Asylum from November 1840 to July 1848; RG5 C1, file 384, Chairman of the Board of Commissioners to the Provincial Secretary, 20 August 1848; Governor General to Provincial Secretary, no date; RG5 C1, file 674, Asylum Commissioners to Provincial Secretary, 12 October 1848; RG5 C1, file 729, Commissioners to Provincial Secretary, 12 March 1849.

50 NA, RG5 C1, file 1492, Report of the Medical Superintendent for 1853; RG5 C1, file 721, Workman to Commissioners 16 June 1854; RG5 C1, file 662, Superintendent's Report, 1856; RG5 C1, file 1232, Workman Report to Commissioners, 5 August 1856; RG5 C1, file 1673, Workman to Commissioners, 4 December 1856; RG5 C1, Report of the Medical Superintendent, 16 January 1867.

51 The establishment of an asylum for the criminally insane at Kingston in 1855 also helped relieve Workman of this "class" of insanity.

52 NA, RG5 C1, Report of the Medical Superintendent, 8 July 1856

53 NA, RG5 C1, file 2235, Superintendent's Report, 3 December 1858

54 The Board of Inspectors of Prisons, Asylums and Public Charities was created as a result of efforts on the part of the united provinces of Canada East and Canada West to systematize and bureaucratize the inspection and control of a range of state institutions. This aspect of state-building deserves its own study, which is beyond the scope of this work.

55 See for example the Annual Report of the Board of Inspectors of Prisons, Asylums and Public Charities, 1862, in *JLA*.

56 NA, RG5 C1, file 223, extract of Minutes of Board of Inspectors in regard to additional Asylum Accommodation, 1 February 1855.

57 Ibid.

58 NA, RG5 C1, file 1063, Deputy Clerk of the Crown to Provincial Secretary, 24 October 1862; copy of Grand Jury Presentment on the State of the Perth Jail; Perth Sheriff to Grand Jury, 12 November 1862

59 NA, RG5 C1, file 1063, Workman to Provincial Secretary, 17 July 1863

60 NA, RG5 C1, file 1063, Taché to Provincial Secretary, 27 July 1863

61 NA, RG5 C1, file 1063, Workman to Provincial Secretary, 5 December 1863

62 NA, RG5 C1, file 106, Petition of the Municipal Council of the Counties of Huron and Bruce, 29 January 1855; RG5 C1, file 305, Petition of the Municipal Council of Wellington, 2 December 1860; RG5 C1, file 1787, Petition of the Waterloo Municipal Council, 22 December 1856. See also RG5 C1, file 1500, Warden of the Stormont and Dundas County Jail to Provincial Secretary, 15 November 1855; RG5 C1, file 120 Chief Justice Draper to Provincial Secretary, 23 April 1859.

63 NA, RG5 C1, file 261, Memorial of the municipal council of the county of Norfolk, 1859

64 NA, RG5 C1, file 127, Chief Justice Robinson to the Provincial Secretary, 22 November 1859; Workman to the Provincial Secretary, 12 December 1859. See also RG5 C1, file 117, Superintendent's Report, 16 January 1857; RG5 C1, file 332, Superintendent's Report on the state of the asylum, 1857.

65 "Sans exprimer une opinion sur les effets spirituels de ces pratiques religieuses ... nous sommes convaincus qu'elles sont très importantes comme moyens curatifs; elles peuvent dominer les idées trop absolues des malades, fixer leur versatilité, et leur inspirer une sage défiance contre leurs propres illusions. Plusieurs de ces patients, turbulents et indisciplinés dans les salles, deviennent, tout à coup, et demeurent pendant le service, silencieux, attentifs et respectueux. Les souvenirs d'autrefois, les coutumes et les sensations du passé revivent et un avantage marqué le résultat." Ibid.

66 Returns from the local jails exist for the years 1856 (the first year that the government originally distributed the circular), 1859, 1860, and 1861. See NA, RG5 C1, files 1677, 518, 857, and 209. The total number of insane reported by the jails for each of these years is a follows: 1856, 35; 1859, 30; 1860, 18; 1861, 27.

67 NA, RG5 C1, file 5801, Petition of the Warden and councillors of the Niagara District, 12 May 1843; RG5 C1, file 6756, Petition of the Warden and Municipal Council of Newcastle, 16 November 1843; RG5 C1, file 7195, Council of the Ottawa District to the Provincial Secretary, 4 February 1844; RG5 C1, file 16160, Warden of the Eastern District to the Provincial Secretary, 1847; RG5 C1, file 5973, Perth Clerk of the Peace to Provincial Secretary, 17 June 1843

68 NA, RG5 C1, file 1039, Warden of Hastings County Jail to the Provincial Secretary, 30 July 1852; RG5 C1, file 1303, Municipal Council of Lincon and Welland to the Provincial Secretary, 1852; RG5 C1, file 1304, Memorial of the Warden and Councillors of the United Counties of Lincoln and Welland for a Reduction of the Lunatic Asylum Tax, 1852. See

also RG5 CI, file 1697, Sheriff of Toronto to Provincial Secretary, 18
October 1852; Solicitor General to Sheriff, 23 October 1852.

69 The warden of the Lincoln and Welland county jail claimed that,
although the average number of their patients looked after in the asylum
was three, the annual tax paid for the support of the institution was
£700. NA, RG5 CI, Warden to Provincial Secretary, 9 November 1855.
See also RG5 CI, file 680, Memorial of the Magistrates of the County of
Norfolk, 9 April 1857.

CHAPTER THREE

1 Recent efforts to marshal and interpret the complex historiography of
the field include Brown, "Dance of the Dialectic?"; Scull, "Psychiatry
and Its Historians"; Mora, "The History of Psychiatry in the United
States."

2 For instance, in her work on eighteenth- and early nineteenth-century
madness, Mary Ann Jiminez traces changing perceptions of, and
responses to, insanity in the United States. With the rise of the lunatic
asylum, however, more traditional forms of management and care fall
away from her historical account. Jiminez, *Changing Faces of Madness*.
A similar approach can be found in Grob's recent synthesis, *The Mad
Among Us*. Despite Cellard's thorough analysis of pre-asylum perceptions and responses to insanity, he demonstrates a similar orientation in
his *Histoire de la folie au Québec*.

3 Tomes, *A Generous Confidence*, 123

4 A similar approach can be found in McCandless, *Moonlight, Magnolias
and Madness*.

5 This was the opinion of Superintendent Workman for the province of
Ontario. See NA, RG5 CI, file 349, Report on the State of the Asylum to
the Visiting Commissioners, 1 March 1854.

6 Prestwich, "Family Strategies and Medical Power," 810

7 For an analysis of non-institutional "customs of community care" in nineteenth-century New Jersey society, see Moran, "Asylum in the Community." See also Bartlett and Wright eds., *Outside the Walls of the Asylum*.

8 In this chapter it will be argued that, contrary to the findings of Tomes,
very little consensus developed between the patrons of the asylum and
asylum superintendents. This difference is perhaps due to the class backgrounds of the patrons and patients of the public asylums of Ontario
and Quebec as compared to those of the patrons and patients of the private Pennsylvania Asylum for the Insane.

9 Wright notes that implicit in many studies of asylum history is the view
that there developed an "uncritical acceptance of medical paradigms of
madness amongst a lay public, as if the non-educated masses would cast

off centuries-old cultural and popular ideas about insanity when confronted by the medical gaze." Wright, "Getting Out of the Asylum," 144.

10 There were, however, four physicians on the Board of Commissioners of the institution. The members of the board were to make regular visits to the asylum.

11 Rules and Regulations of the Montreal Lunatic Asylum

12 For instance, male patients under attendant supervision chopped wood for the asylum. Cellard and Nadon assume that female patients' work included various domestic duties. There is no evidence for this but it would reflect prevailing asylum wisdom. Cellard and Nadon, "Ordre et désordre," 359

13 Rules and Regulations of the Montreal Lunatic Asylum

14 The asylum was also equipped with patient day rooms and refectories. See Cellard and Nadon's physical description of the asylum in "Ordre et désordre," 358.

15 NA, RG4 B65, file 1731, John Boston and J. Trestler to Governor General, 23 August 1843

16 NA, RG4 B65, file 2812, Statement of the Number of Lunatics Admitted to the Montreal Lunatic Asylum from November 1839 to July 31 1844, and How Disposed With

17 NA, RG4 B65, Miscellaneous Documents, Medical Report of Dr Rees to the Commissioners, 1 September 1844

18 Rees's treatment methods can be pieced together from the following documents: NA, RG5 C1, file 8870, Report of the Board of Physicians for Inspecting the Temporary Lunatic Asylum at Toronto, Report of Dr Joseph Hamilton, 9 October 1844; Report of Dr Beaumont, no date; Report of Dr Walter Telfer, 14 October 1844. RG5 C1, file 602, Report of Dr Spears, 17 March 1843. See also the medical records from Rees's prescription book in RG5 C1, file 8870.

19 NA, RG4 B65, Miscellaneous Documents, Rees's Medical Report, 1844

20 Bynum notes that Broussais's "treatment of choice for virtually all diseases was leeching, which, he argued, produced counter-irritation and reduction of the inflammatory origin of the process." See Bynum, "Nosology," 350. See also Prichard, *A Treatise on Insanity and Other Disorders Affecting the Mind*.

21. See for example Rush's instructions for cases of mania, which included bloodletting, cupping, low diet, and the use of cold in *Medical Inquiries and Observations upon the Diseases of the Mind*, 190–9. Rees did not adhere to Rush's use of calomel in such cases.

22 NA, RG5 C1, file 242, Medical Report of Dr Primrose, 31 December 1849. See also RG5 C1, file 13434, Annual Report of Superintendent Telfer, 1845; RG5 C1, Report of Superintendent Primrose, 2 April 1849

23 Annual Report of Superintendent Walter Telfer, 1847; Report of Superintendent Primrose, 25 January 1850

24 See Stephenson, "Medicine and Architecture," 1505–8.

25 In the 1852 attack, 25 cases of cholera in the asylum were reported, 13 of which resulted in death. NA, RG5 C1, file 1813, Chairman of the Board of Commissioners to Provincial Secretary, 8 November 1852; Superintendent Scott's Report, 6 December 1852.

26 NA, RG5 C1, file 1966, Minutes from the Board of Directors on the State of the Asylum, 6 December 1852

27 NA, RG5 C1, file 199, Report of Professor Croft on Ventilation; Report on the Drainage and Water Supply, 11 February 1853. RG4 C1, file 43, John Howard to Provincial Secretary, 4 January 1853

28 NA, RG5 C1, file 1492, Report of the Medical Superintendent, 20 September 1853

29 NA, RG5 C1, Report of the Medical Superintendent, 20 September 1853; Supplementary Report, 1 October 1853

30 NA, RG5 C1, file 1812, Report of the Superintendent on the State of the Asylum, 20 October 1853

31 Ibid.

32 Report of the Medical Superintendent, 20 September 1853; Supplementary Report, 1 October 1853. For a fuller discussion of miasmata and its socio-medical origins, see Hannaway, "Environment and Miasmata."

33 NA, RG5 C1, file 1812, Report on the State of the Asylum, 20 October 1853. The patients were set to work as a labour-saving measure. Wanting to make the connection between the asylum environment and insanity clear to the commissioners, Workman noted that one convalescent patient employed in such work suffered a temporary relapse of insanity.

34 He tried to correct this air deficiency by cutting holes in the roof of the asylum and in the walls between rooms.

35 For a sample of the many reports in which Workman complains of overcrowding, see NA, RG5 C1, file 349, Report on the State of the Asylum, 1 March 1854; RG5 C1, file 489, Report of the Medical Superintendent, 14 April 1854; RG5 C1, file 755, Annual Report of the Medical Superintendent, 1854.

36 NA, RG5 C1, file 589, Report of the Medical Superintendent, 5 April 1855

37 NA, RG5 C1, file 608, Report of the Medical Superintendent, 9 May 1854; and RG5 C1, file 755, Annual Report of the Medical Superintendent, 1854. See also RG5 C1, file 1232, Report of the Medical Superintendent, 5 August 1856; RG5 C1, file 1673, Workman to the Provincial Secretary, 4 December 1856. Workman went so far as to blame the lack of means for classification for a case of suicide in the asylum. See RG5 C1, file 2007, Report of the Medical Superintendent, 18 October 1858. Workman's frustration about overcrowding increased with the passing of an act in 1851 for the removal of the criminally insane from the Kingston Penitentiary to

the Toronto Asylum. As lunatics of the "criminal class" began filtering into the institution from the penitentiary, Workman became even more convinced of the therapeutic deficiencies resulting from the lack of proper patient classification at the Toronto Asylum.

38 Although the London Asylum certainly did not reproduce the environmental disaster that befell the Toronto Asylum in its first six years, S.E.D. Shortt notes that "despite both the grand exterior of the asylum, the largest building in the western half of the province, and the best intentions of the architect from the Public Works Department, the [London Asylum] was plagued with organizational and structural problems from its inception." Shortt, *Victorian Lunacy*, 29

39 For Canada, see especially the discussion of degeneration theory in Shortt, ibid., ch. 4, "The Social Genesis of Etiological Speculation."

40 *Rapport aux Commissaires de L'Asyle Temporaire des Aliénés, à Beauport*, janvier 1849

41 NA, RG4 B65, file 2423, Report of Douglas, Morrin and Frémont, 16 September 1852; RG4 B65, Report of the Commissioner of the Beauport Asylum, 27 April 1850. In 1863 a new asylum with a central building and two wings was again constructed, incorporating further improvements.

42 See, for example, NA, RG4 B65, file 2392, "Copie de quelques remarques faites par le médecin visiteur sur l'Asile des Aliénés à Beauport," 6 October to 30 October 1865. See also RG4 B65, file 1809, Report of Visiting Physician Dr A. Jackson on the Beauport Lunatic Asylum to Provincial Secretary, 18 September 1866; Jackson Report to Provincial Secretary, 7 January 1867; Provincial Secretary to Secretary to the Commissioners of the Beauport Lunatic Asylum, 18 January 1867; Jackson to N.F. Belham, 21 February 1867.

43 Report of the Royal Commission on Lunatic Asylums of the Province of Quebec, *1888*, 49–50. Some caution must be used when evaluating the findings of the Royal Commission. Part of the commissioners' critique of Beauport was related to their agenda of converting the institution into a less expensive enterprise under the auspices of religious charity. To this end the Commissioners juxtaposed the defects of the Beauport Asylum with the efficiency and cleanliness of Saint-Jean-de-Dieu. But in the opinion of Daniel Tuke, who evaluated the asylums of Canada on a tour in 1884, Saint-Jean-de-Dieu was by far the worst asylum in the two provinces. See Tuke, *The Insane in the United States and Canada*.

44 Report of the Commissioners Appointed to Superintend the Beauport Lunatic Asylum, 1855, *Quebec Sessional Papers*, 19 Vict. Appendix no. 2, 1856

45 See the dramatic description of events in the 1875 Report of the Quebec Lunatic Asylum by the Medical Superintendents, *Sessional Papers*, 38 Vict., No. 26, 1874–75.

46 See Burgess, "A Historical Sketch," 71.

47 NA, RG5 C1, file 1492, Report of the Medical Superintendent of the Toronto Asylum, 20 September 1853

48 Beauport's house surgeon noted of work therapy that "all who have studied this subject agree in acknowledging its immense importance not only with respect to bodily health and good order, but also as one of the most efficacious therapeutic agents in the treatment of insanity." Report of the House Surgeon of the Lunatic Asylum at Beauport, *Sessional Papers*, 27 Vict., No. 39, 1864. Workman noted to the commissioners with satisfaction that upwards of three-fifths of his patient population worked at various tasks.

49 Report of the Quebec Lunatic Asylum by the Medical Superintendents, 1872–73, *Sessional Papers*, 37 Vict., No. 5, 1873, 114

50 NA, RG5 C1, file 1492, Supplementary Report of the Medical Superintendent, 1 October 1853. Superintendent Roy of the Beauport Asylum put it this way: "Manual labour ... fortifies the physical organisation of the patient and largely contributes to the maintenance of order and the preservation of the morals of the patient." 1872–73 Report of the Quebec Lunatic Asylum by the Medical Superintendents, *Sessional Papers*, Vict. 37, No. 5, 1873.

51 NA, RG4 B65, Petition for the Release of Jean Dupont from the Beauport Lunatic Asylum, 28 August 1849; Provincial Secretary to Commissioners of the Beauport Lunatic Asylum, 10 September 1849. The petition was sent during the construction of the new asylum at La Canardière.

52 Annual Report of the Proprietors of the Beauport Lunatic Asylum, 1869, *Sessional Papers*, 34 Vict. No. 12, 1870

53 *Archives of Ontario*, (hereafter AO), RG 63, Correspondence of the Inspector of Prisons and Private Charities (hereafter IC), file 6387, Christie to Provincial Secretary, 22 February 1894

54 AO, RG 63, IC, file 6387, Clark to Christie, 20 February 1894

55 AO, RG 63, IC, file 2387, Christie to Provincial Secretary, 22 February 1894

56 See for example Christie's efforts to save money in this way with the use of supervised patient labour in the asylum bakery, AO, RG 63, IC, file 6370, Christie to Clark, 3 July 1895.

57 See Steward's Report in the Annual Report of the Malden Asylum, 1868–69.

58 AO, RG 63, IC, file 6391, Clark to Christie, 2 December 1895. See also Christie's recommendation of Mr McCammon for the position of asylum baker, AO, RG 63, IC, file 6370, Christie to Clark, 15 May 1895.

59 Report of Dr Wolfred Nelson, *Sessional Papers*, 25 Vict., No. 19, 1862

60 Thus Workman noted in an annual report that "the coats of the male patients alone have last year been made out of the asylum. All other

needlework has been done in the house by the female patients, and some
males directed by a jobbing tailor." Shortly after his appointment as
superintendent to the Malden Asylum, Henry Landor noted that "no
one in charge of any asylum can lay a greater stress on the necessity of
[patient] employment than myself." John Palmer Litchfield, superintendent of the Rockwood Criminal Lunatic Asylum, noted that the value of
the labour of many of his patients cannot well be questioned. One of
them cooks all the food required for the male inmates of the Asylum,
another supplies it to those who cannot serve themselves ... [another]
fabricates the warm clothing required to keep them in health, and ...
[another] nurses them tenderly in sickness, and closes their eyes reveren-
tially when they die." See Report of the Rockwood Criminal Lunatic
Asylum for 1866, *Journals of the Legislative Assembly of Upper Canada*
(hereafter *JLAUC*)

61   See for example, NA, RG5 C1, file 570, Workman's Report on the State of
the Asylum, 18 March 1858. Although the Beauport proprietors did not
give such statistical returns, they had by far the largest institutional farm
under production in Canada, comprising some 200 acres. The farm at
the Toronto Asylum was 30 acres in size. Superintendents placed a heavy
emphasis on the productivity of patients at the Malden and Orillia
Branch Asylums, as is reflected in these institutions' annual reports. For
Malden, see Annual Report of Superintendent Fisher, 1862, *Sessional
Papers*, 66; and the annual reports for 1863, 1864, and 1865. For Orillia, see Annual Report of Superintendent Ardagh, 1862, *Sessional
Papers*, no 66; and the annual reports for 1863, 1864, 1865, and 1866.
Patient work was also of great importance during the renovations of the
branch asylums in Ontario. Workman noted, for example, that on 14
July 1859, "twenty of our most industrious and quiet male patients
[were sent to the Malden Asylum] to assist in the works to be performed." Annual Report of the Superintendent, 1859. Two years later,
Workman praised Superintendent Fisher of the Malden Asylum for "his
skill in the direction of the labour of his patients," which helped save
"the public much expense in the preparation of the buildings and
premises." Annual Report of Superintendent Workman, 1860.

62   See AO, RG63, Box 229, file 6595, Inspector Aerial to Bucke, 12 March
1883; Bucke to Aerial, 31 March 1883; Bucke to Aerial, 29 March
1884; Aerial to Bucke, 30 January 1884; Bucke to Aerial, 18 February
1884; Aerial to Bucke, 20 February 1884; Bucke to Aerial, 28 February
1884; Aerial to Bucke, 4 March 1884; Provincial Secretary to Bucke, 10
March 1884. Maurice Bucke of the London Asylum was especially concerned with creating new forms of work for his patients. In 1884 Bucke
managed to get 84 per cent of his 900 patients to work "on an average
day." To increase the number of patients working at the asylum, he gave

extra privileges to those who worked and withheld the privileges of those who did not. See Shortt, *Victorian Lunacy*, 132. Bucke introduced the cultivation of willows for basket making and the manufacturing of bed mattresses in an effort to increase and diversify the productivity of his patient labour force at the asylum.

63   Soon after his permanent appointment, Workman had a planked walkway constructed by patient labour, in order that patients could take walks around the asylum grounds without getting wet from the damp soil.

64   At Beauport the proprietors subscribed to the *Bibliothèque de Québec* for books for patients. At the Toronto Asylum, the first library was established from books selected by Workman himself.

65   Annual Report of the Beauport Proprietors, Quebec, 1849

66   Shortt, *Victorian Lunacy*, 136

67   By 1854 Workman estimated that three-fifths of his patient population were "hopeless" cases. NA, RG5 C1, file 755, Annual Report of the Medical Superintendent.

68   See Report of the Medical Proprietors of the Beauport Asylum, 13 December 1855, *Sessional Papers*, 19 Vict., Appendix 2. See also NA, RG5 C1, file 1673, Workman to the Provincial Secretary, 4 December 1856.

69   Report of the House Surgeon of the Lunatic Asylum at Beauport, 28 January 1864, *Sessional Papers*, 27 Vict., No. 39, 1864. See also Report of the Quebec Lunatic Asylum by the Medical Superintendents, 1872–73, *Sessional Papers*, Vict. 37, No. 5, 42; Annual Report of the Proprietors of the Beauport Lunatic Asylum for the Year 1869, *Sessional Papers*, 34 Vict., No. 12, 1870, 43

70   NA, RG5 C1, file 1243, Report of the Superintendent, 1854. In an attempt to remedy this perceived evil, Workman offered to give a series of lectures on "insanity and the bodily disorders associated with it" at the asylum for the benefit of students at Toronto medical schools.

71   NA, RG5 C1, file 720, Report of the Medical Superintendent, 3 May 1855. Workman argued that "the most promising [asylum] cases are generally those for which the least has been done" by the local physician. NA, RG4 C1, file 332, Report on the State of the Asylum, 1857. Lamenting the average physician's lack of education in psychiatry, Superintendent Roy states: "They understand what they have learned, but they were not taught everything that was necessary for the future; thus, when called to attend a patient, they cannot sometimes analyze, at once, the symptoms of mental alienation or of a nervous disease, where it exists; they direct all their attention to the patient, and try correctly to see their way through the doubts which they entertain, but notwithstanding their watchfulness and good intentions, the disease becomes

more serious; the latest period, being the precursor of delirium is passed, unnoticed by them, frenzy suddenly and most unexpectedly supervenes, and then all is clear ... but it is too late." Report of the Quebec Lunatic Asylum by the Medical Superintendents, 1872–3, *Sessional Papers*, Vict. 37, No. 5, 119–20.

72 See for example, Annual Report of the Proprietors of the Beauport Lunatic Asylum for the Year 1869, *Sessional Papers*, 34 Vict., No. 12, 1870, 44; Report of the Quebec Lunatic Asylum by the Medical Superintendents, 1872–73, *Sessional Papers*, Vict. 37, No.5, 47.

73 See, NA, RG5 C1, file 608, Report of the Medical Superintendent, 9 May 1854.

74 The superintendents in Quebec appeared to exclude the religious hospitals in Quebec, including the Montreal General Hospital, the House of Providence in Montreal, the Montreal Lying-In Hospital, and the Quebec General Hospital, from their castigations. The insane were frequently sent to these charitable institutions as a first resort in the hopes that medical treatment there would result in recovery. But as soon as the patients' behaviour became intractable to the point of disrupting the medical regimen of the other patients, the Sisters refused to keep them. A petition was usually then sent to have the patient removed to the Beauport Lunatic Asylum. See, NA, RG4 C1, file 1471; RG4 C1, file 2784; RG4 C1, file 1790; RG4 C1, file 1601; RG4 C1, file 3223; RG4 C1, file 1990; RG4 C1, file 1423; RG4 C1, file 350; RG4 C1, file 1210; RG4 C1, file 1276; RG4 C1, file 1605; RG4 C1, file 1607; RG4 C1, file 2304; RG4 C1, file 696; RG4 C1, file 701; RG4 C1, file 1415.

75 For instance, at the Midland District Jail a physician was hired to "make quarterly reports on the health of the prisoners and the several cases of sickness which have occurred with the term just ended. For his services he is allowed a compensation of fifty pounds per annum – and though engaged for the benefit of the inmates of the cells only, he never hesitates to extend his professional aid to unfortunate and penniless debtors when required." See Midland District Gaol Report, Kingston, 30 December 1835, *JLA*. Appendix #44, 1836. See also London District Gaol Report, London, 31 December 1835, *JLA*.

76 This examination is based on the correspondence between the clerk of the peace of the Perth County Jail and the superintendent of the Toronto Lunatic Asylum. See, AO, RG 22, Clerk of the Peace, Lunatic Accounts, Perth County, unprocessed (hereafter, Lunatic Accounts, Perth County).

77 AO, Lunatic Accounts, Perth County, Clerk of the Peace to Joseph Workman, 30 July 1858

78 AO, Lunatic Accounts, Perth County, Questionnaire for the Committal of Patricia Peters, April 1858. Hyde treated another patient who was suffering from a condition that appeared to the surgeon to be "more like

nervous fever than pure insanity" with wine freely laced with opiates and occasionally (owing to the unhealthy evacuations) with calomel. See Questionnaire for the Committal of John Lang, 15 June 1860.

79 AO, Lunatic Accounts, Perth County, Dr Hyde to Linton, 2 August 1860; Linton to Workman, 9 August 1860

80 AO, Lunatic Accounts, Perth County, Workman to Linton, 11 June 1860

81 AO, Lunatic Accounts, Perth County, Workman to Linton, 18 June 1860. Hyde was evidently not one of those country physicians whose unenlightened treatment strategies were so lamented by Workman and other alienists. The success of the jail surgeon could determine who was to be sent to the asylum. For example, at the London Jail in 1865, applications were made for two lunatics to be sent to the asylum. But a short time later the sheriff wrote to the provincial secretary stating that one of the patients had "improved greatly under the treatment of the jail physician – If you find you have only room for one, I would much rather send you [the other], as he is very violent, and difficult to manage." NA, RG5 C1, file 1038, Sheriff to Provincial Secretary, 29 July 1865

82 AO, Lunatic Accounts, Perth County, Linton to Workman, 27 February 1858; Hyde to Linton, 8 March 1858

83 AO, Lunatic Accounts, Perth County, Linton to Workman, 12 April 1858

84 AO, Lunatic Accounts, Perth County, Workman to Linton, 10 May 1858

85 AO, Lunatic Accounts, Perth County, John Sparling to Linton, 6 May 1858; Linton to John Sparling, J.P., 27 May 1858

86 AO, Lunatic Accounts, Perth County, R. McDonnell to Linton, 23 December 1858

87 AO, Lunatic Accounts, Perth County, Linton to Workman, 15 July 1858; Linton to Workman, 16 July 1858

88 AO, Lunatic Accounts, Perth County, Linton to Workman, 20 August 1858

89 AO, Lunatic Accounts, Perth County, Calvin Collins to Linton, 20 September 1859; Linton to Collins, 20 September 1859

90 AO, Lunatic Accounts, Perth County, Collins to Linton, 19 October 1859

91 AO, Lunatic Accounts, Perth County, Hyde to Linton, 21 June 1860

92 AO, Lunatic Accounts, Perth County, Collins to Linton, 2 July 1860; Linton to Collins, 4 July 1860

93 Linton likewise kept ongoing correspondence with the asylum superintendent on the condition of patients sent from the local jail. See, for example, the correspondence between Mrs Foster, Linton, and the superintendent on the progress of Foster's husband. AO, Lunatic Accounts, Perth County, 8 June 1853.

94 See for example NA, RG4 C1, file 801, Beaubien to Provincial Secretary, 7 May 1851.

95 See for example NA, RG4 C1, file 564, Report of the Jail Surgeon, 2 April 1851.

96 Indeed, the obvious advantages of having alienist and jail physician as one and the same prompted fellow proprietor Dr Frémont to apply for the position of physician to the Quebec Jail during Morrin's leave of absence in 1857. Frémont was late in applying to be the replacement, however, and despite a personal and friendly appeal to the government the position was given to Drs Nault and Roy. See NA, RG4 C1, Frémont to Taché, 3 June 1857; Provincial Secretary to Frémont, 8 June 1857.

97 See for example the speedy committal of a male patient from the Quebec Jail to the asylum in NA, RG4 C1, file 1270, Joseph Morrin to Provincial Secretary, 18 June 1852.

98 See NA, RG4 C1, file 1967, Morrin to Provincial Secretary, 18 October 1853; Provincial Secretary to Morrin, 19 October 1853, where Morrin notes that one of his patients, for whom a warrant was issued for removal to the asylum, had in the interim, been "taken care of by his friends." For a similar case, see NA, RG4 C1, Sheriff of the Sherbrooke Jail to Provincial Secretary, 28 January 1861; Sheriff to the Provincial Secretary, 2 February 1861.

99 NA, RG4 C1, file 863, Petition for the Committal of Jean Dubois, 1856.

100 The deplorable conditions of some local jails did not lend themselves to any amelioration of the conditions of lunatics incarcerated there, regardless of the presence or absence of medical treatment. See for example NA, RG5 C1, file 1525, Presentment of the Grand Jury, 16 November 1854; Presentment of the Grand Jury, 20 October 1854, and especially, RG5 C1, file 1856, Sheriff of Cobourg to Provincial Secretary, 11 April 1856; Grand Jury Presentment, 9 April 1856.

101 See for example Connor, "'A Sort of Felo-De-Se'"; Gidney and Miller, "Origins of Organized Medicine in Ontario."

102 "Sa maladie pourrait peut-être se guérir, s'il était confiné dans un asyle et soumis à un traitement tandis que continuant à demeurer au milieu de sa famille on ne peut s'attendre à un dernier résultat, ainsi que l'expérience nous l'enseigne." NA, RG4 C1, file 422, Medical Certificate of Dr Charles [surname illegible], 1 February 1867

103 "La maladie menace [de] devenir chronique et incurable, tandis que placé dans un hospice, ce jeune homme aurait toutes les chances d'une guérisson prompte et durable sous les soins [des] personnes de l'asile." NA, RG4 C1, file 142, Medical Certificate of Dr Proulx, 19 January 1858. For other examples, see NA, RG4 C1, file 1379, Medical Certificate of Dr David, 16 May 1855. See also RG4 C1, file 1566, Medical Certificate of Dr J.M. Dechêne of St Anne de la Patière, 4 July 1859; RG4 C1, file 880, Medical Certificate of Dr F. Gilbert of Hatley East Township, 5 May 1853.

104 "La simple justice pour cette section du pays, et ses besoins locaux,

demandent un semblable établissement à celui de Beauport." NA, RG4 CI, file 1890, Medical Certificate of Dr Gerand, 16 September 1859.

105 NA, RG4 CI, file 708, J.D. Laurendeau, médecin de St Gabriel de Brandou to Provincial Secretary, 11 May 1854; Laurendeau to Provincial Secretary, 13 July 1854

106 NA, RG4 CI, file 838, Medical Certificate of Dr M.S. Scott, 13 June 1859

107 See NA, RG4 CI, file 1411, Physician's Medical Certificate, 1856; RG4 CI, file 1737, Dr David to Provincial Secretary, 9 September 1853

108 Nevertheless, as in Ontario, during periods of institutional overcrowding, Beauport's strategy was to admit only recent, curable cases.

109 Dr Gilbert of Hatley Eastern Township thus noted that a patient "has for some months been gradually getting worse and I see no prospect of his ever being any better. He is now quite dangerous having attempted the lives of several persons and threatened to destroy himself ... Under these circumstances I believe it is the province of Government to place the party in an asylum." NA, RG4 CI, file 2614, Dr Gilbert to Provincial Secretary, 25 October 1852

110 NA, RG4 CI, file 30, Medical Certificate of Dr John Fitzpatrick, 6 January 1854

111 NA, RG4 CI, file 2030, Medical Certificate of Dr Wolfred Nelson, 19 June 1849

112 NA, RG4 CI, file 1098, Dr Paquin to Provincial Secretary, 3 June 1853; Paquin to Provincial Secretary, 4 July 1853. See also NA, RG4 CI, file 2403 for a doctor's concerns about the social repercussions of the nymphomaniacal symptoms of his patient's insanity. Also, NA, RG4 CI, file 1959, Medical Certificate, 25 May 1848; RG4 CI, file 1134, Medical Certificate of Dr L.M. Bardy, 7 June 1853

113 Jacalyn Duffin, *Langstaff: A Nineteenth-Century Medical Life*, 127

114 Ibid., 131–8.

CHAPTER FOUR

1 This was a time of financial uncertainty for the Toronto Asylum when the commissioners had decided to take the drastic measure of temporarily prohibiting the entry of pauper patients.

2 NA, RG5 CI, file 1535, James Hardey to Provincial Secretary, 21 September 1852; Provincial Secretary to Hardey, 27 September 1852

3 NA, RG5 CI, file 1852, Hardey to Provincial Secretary, 15 October 1852

4 For examples of wealthier families' motivations for committal see Tomes, *A Generous Confidence*, 90–128; Warsh, *Moments of Unreason*, 63–81; Prestwich, "Family Strategies and Medical Power." On pauper families and the context of committal see Walton, "Casting Out

and Bringing Back in Victorian England." Mitchinson assesses motivations for committal to the Toronto Asylum in, Mitchinson, "Reasons for Committal to a Mid-Nineteenth-Century Ontario Insane Asylum."

5 Wright, "Getting Out of the Asylum," 144.

6 Finnane, "Asylums, Families and the State," 135, quoted in Wright, ibid., 143.

7 See NA, RG4 C1, file 1037, Provincial Secretary to Reverend John Cornwall, 27 May 1850. See also RG4 C1, file 2350, 1850.

8 NA, RG4 C1, file 1990, J.R. Ecrement, JP, to Provincial Secretary, 15 October 1854; Provincial Secretary to Ecrement, 9 October 1854; Reverend Anderson to Provincial Secretary, 14 August 1854

9 NA, RG4 C1, file 1367, Reverend W. Anderson to Provincial Secretary, 8 August 1854; Provincial Secretary to Anderson, 12 August 1854; Medical Certificate of Dr E.W. Carter, 12 August 1854. For a similar example, see NA, RG4 C1, file 2657.

10 NA, RG4 C1, Carlisle to Provincial Secretary, 20 August 1853

11 The phrase is borrowed from Parr, *The Gender of Breadwinners*.

12 NA, RG4 C1, file 3079, Petition of Margaret Bennett, 28 October 1848; Provincial Secretary to Bennett, 4 November 1848. A remarkably similar example of two needleworkers whose widowed mother becomes insane can be found in NA, RG4 C1, file 1570.

13 NA, RG4 C1, file 2052, Petition of Abraham Deignault, 22 October 1851. See also RG4 C1, file 1688, 1859.

14 NA, RG4 C1, file 1113, Roman Catholic Bishop of Montreal to Provincial Secretary, 5 July 1854; Medical Certificate of Dr Louis Giard, 24 June 1854. The use of the orphanage in Quebec as part of the survival strategy for poor families is discussed in Bradbury, *Working Families*, 208–10.

15 NA, RG5 C1, file 2120, Petition of William Noel of the town of Niagara, 8 November 1841

16 NA, RG4 C1, file 1985, Petition of G. Johnston, 21 October 1853

17 See for example NA, RG4 C1, file 3300; RG4 C1, file 3086; RG4 C1, file 1227; RG4 C1, file 3139

18 NA, RG4 C1, file 2613, Petition of the Residents of St Catherine, 28 October 1852

19 See for example, NA, RG4 C1, file 2129; RG4 C1, file 2850; RG4 C1, file 1697.

20 NA, RG4 C1, file 3236, Célestin Déry to Provincial Secretary, 3 December 1845; Petition of the Inhabitants of Quebec, 4 December 1845. See also RG4 C1, file 1506, Father L.T. Bernard to Provincial Secretary, 22 June 1857; RG4 C1, file 2090, Petition of the Inhabitants of Lachine, 26 June 1849.

21 NA, RG4 C1, file 148, Bishop of Quebec to Provincial Secretary, 23 January 1857. See also RG4 C1, file 430.

22 NA, RG4 C1, file 2265, Langevin to Provincial Secretary, 13 August 1856;
    RG4 C1, file 1981, L. Massue to Provincial Secretary, 21 October 1853
23 See for example NA, RG5 C1, file 1944, Sheriff of Cornwall to Provincial
    Secretary, 3 October 1849; RG5 C1, file 147, Sheriff of Cornwall to
    Provincial Secretary, 2 February 1849
24 "Je supporte ces enfants depuis un grand nombre d'années et n'ai
    jamais voulu les placer à l'asile de Beauport, ou du moins demander
    une place pour eux malgré l'état de pauvreté dans lequel je me trou-
    vais. Mais aujourdhui je suis pauvre et avancé en âge; de plus mon
    épouse sur laquelle je comptais pour veiller avec soin sur ces enfants
    est maintenant malade, âgée et incapable de s'acquitter de cette tâche
    penible de sorte que je suis obligé de vous supplier d'accorder une
    place pour mes deux enfants à l'asile de Beauport avec pension." NA,
    RG4 C1, file 2121, Philipe Proux to Provincial Secretary, 6 August
    1862
25 NA, RG4 C1, file 1679, Magé to Provincial Secretary, 20 July 1859
26 NA, RG4 C1, file 2819, Woods to Provincial Secretary, 17 March 1851.
    See also RG4 C1, file 2861; file 1817; and file 2244.
27 NA, RG4 C1, file 1371, Massé to Provincial Secretary, 27 April 1848
28 NA, RG4 C1, file 1650, Mignault to Provincial Secretary, 10 June 1855
29 NA, RG4 C1, file 402, Laurent to Provincial Secretary, 19 February 1862.
    See also RG4 C1, file 552.
30 See for example NA, file 2240, Paré to Provincial Secretary, 10 Novem-
    ber 1854, for the case of a man considered to be both violent and
    embarrassing in his behaviour. See also RG4 C1, file 1190. The social
    unease resulting from the onset of aberrant behaviour among servants in
    nineteenth-century Canadian society could also form grounds for com-
    mittal by their employers. See for example, NA, RG4 C1, file 743, 1854;
    RG4 C1, file 16, 1853; RG4 C1, file 1162, 1852.
31 NA, RG4 C1, file 2235, T. Brodeur to Provincial Secretary, 6 November
    1854
32 NA, RG4 C1, file 2654, Olivier Stream to Provincial Secretary, 3 Novem-
    ber 1852; Petition of the Residents of St Michel d'Yamaska, 1 November
    1852. For another, more fragmentary, example of an abandoned woman
    considered to be insane, see NA, RG4 C1, file 1520, 1851.
33 NA, RG4 C1, file 1745, O'Grady to Provincial Secretary, 20 August 1851.
    For a similar example of a man who was considered "bereft of his rea-
    son," and wandered about annoying the "neighbours every night with
    his shouts and wild noises," see NA, RG4 C1, file 1588, Petition to
    Provincial Secretary, 23 July 1851.
34 NA, RG4 C1, file 1287, Tardif to Provincial Secretary, 23 May 1859
35 NA, RG5 C1, file 10750, McGillivray to James M. Higgmom Esq., 10
    June 1845; Provincial Secretary to McGillivray, 17 June 1845

36 NA, RG4 C1, file 1959, Petition of the Inhabitants of Terrebonne, 25 May 1848. See also RG4 C1, file 2021, 1849.

37 NA, RG4 C1, file 88, Brethor to Provincial Secretary, 13 January 1849. Patients who successfully escaped from the asylums of Ontario and Quebec could, if not quickly recovered, also engage in prolonged periods of "wandering" about the country. See for example NA, RG4 C1, file 1188, John Rose to Provincial Secretary, 17 April 1858; Report of a Committee of the Executive Council, 22 April 1858. See also, RG4 C1, file 757, 1854.

38 NA, RG5 C1, file 18, George Hughes to John McLennan, 26 June 1848; A. Fraser to Provincial Secretary, 7 July 1848. A similar example can be found in RG5 C1, file 874, 1849.

39 NA, RG4 C1, file 1482, Stevenson to Provincial Secretary, 10 July 1851; Provincial Secretary to Stevenson, 22 June 1852; Stevenson to Provincial Secretary, 2 July 1852. See also RG4 C1, file 964, 1853, for a case in which "L'individu en question devenu plus traitable depuis que j'ai fait application pour lui, sa famille s'est décidé à différer encore quelque temps son départ pour l'asile des insensés."

40 NA, RG4 C1, Prayer of Thomas Nelson Yeoman of the Township of Grenville, 8 April 1852; Provincial Secretary to Nelson, 15 April 1852; Provincial Secretary to Nelson, 5 October 1852; Charles Forest (on behalf of Nelson) to Provincial Secretary, 15 October 1852. See also NA, RG4 C1, file 2525, 1852.

41 See for example NA, RG4 C1, file 1520, Dr H. Brown to Provincial Secretary, 17 February 1852.

42 NA, RG4 C1, file 269, Catholic Bishop of Montreal to Provincial Secretary, 14 February 1853; Fakey to Provincial Secretary, 12 March 1853; Provincial Secretary to Fakey, 15 March 1853; Fakey to Provincial Secretary, 16 June 1853.

43 Ibid.

44 NA, RG4 C1, file 708, Dr J.D. Laurendeau to Provincial Secretary, 11 May 1854; Provincial Secretary to Laurendeau, 11 July 1854; Laurendeau to Provincial Secretary, 13 July 1854.

45 NA, RG4 C1, Reverend King to Provincial Secretary, 11 November 1850; Provincial Secretary to King, 15 November 1850; Provincial Secretary to King, 23 December 1850; King to Provincial Secretary, 11 January 1851; Provincial Secretary to King, 13 February 1851; King to Provincial Secretary, 25 March 1851.

46 See for example NA, RG4 C1, where James Douglas noted that a patient "who was admitted on 29 January, 1863, is improved – but not recovered. She is violent and disposed to be distracted when excited. The husband is desirous to obtain her discharge." See also NA, RG4 C1, file 1749, 1854.

47   NA, RG4 C1, file 238, A. Pinsonneault to Provincial Secretary, 12 February 1867; L. Fortin to Provincial Secretary, 8 February 1867; Superintendent Henry Howard to Provincial Secretary, 18 February 1867

48   NA, RG4 C1, file 2037, Martin to Provincial Secretary, 20 June 1849

49   See for example NA, RG4 C1, file 969, 1857; RG4 C1, file 483, 1854; RG4 C1, file 2850, 1852; RG4 C1, file 1915, 1850.

50   NA, RG4 C1, file 3036, Charles Duncan to Provincial Secretary, 12 November 1855; Provincial Secretary to Duncan, 20 November 1855, Duncan to Provincial Secretary, 8 October 1856; RG4 C1, Duncan to Provincial Secretary, 23 June 1857; Provincial Secretary to Duncan, 27 June 1857

51   NA, RG4 C1, file 2294, Reverend Gingras to Provincial Secretary, 12 November 1854; Gingras to Bolduc, 18 December 1854; Chairman of the Commissioners of the Beauport Asylum to Provincial Secretary, 19 December 1854

52   NA, RG4 C1, file 222, Moïse Legault to Provincial Secretary, 11 February 1867; Provincial Secretary to Henry Howard, 12 February 1867; Howard to Provincial Secretary, 14 February 1867; Provincial Secretary to Legault, 18 February 1867

53   A version of this response is found on most rejected petitions.

54   "L'aliéné ... est dans la dernière pauvreté avec une nombreuse famille. Sa femme est dans une affreuse misère et tous leurs parents sont pauvres. C'est au nom de la paroisse que je vous adresse ces lignes. S'il y a moyen de l'admettre dans l'asile, oh! tâchez de le faire. Jamais vous n'aurez rendu un plus grand service à une famille désolée." NA, RG4 C1, file 1098, Dr Paquin to Provincial Secretary, 3 June 1853

55   NA, RG4 C1, file 1098, Medical Certificate of Drs Pillet and Forbes, 3 June 1853; Petition of Inhabitants of St Genevière, 3 June 1853; Paquin to Provincial Secretary, 20 June 1853; Provincial Secretary to Paquin, 22 June 1853; Paquin to Provincial Secretary, 4 July 1853; Provincial Secretary to Paquin, 15 August 1853. Other cases rejected by the government as incurable include: NA, RG4 C1, file 1737, 1853; RG4 C1, file 1411, 1853; RG4 C1, file 1134, 1853; RG4 C1, file 1063, 1853.

56   NA, RG4 C1, file 1885, E.W. Carter to Provincial Secretary, 3 October 1853; Provincial Secretary to Carter, 18 October 1853; Carter to Provincial Secretary, 19 October 1853; Provincial Secretary to Commissioners of the Beauport Lunatic Asylum, 20 October 1853; Provincial Secretary to Carter, 20 October 1853. This patient, like several others in which "probational" status was given, was reported on by the superintendent after the end of the trial period as "improved" but not cured. The government responded by placing her on the permanent list of government patients. For similar cases with the same resolution see NA, RG4 C1, file 1494, 1853; RG4 C1, file 652, 1853.

57 NA, RG4 CI, file 2054, Joseph Dupont to Provincial Secretary, 6 October 1853; Provincial Secretary to Justice of the Peace of St Denis, 7 January 1854

58 NA, RG4 CI, file 1558, Medical Certificate of Dr Morrin, 10 August 1853

59 NA, RG4 CI, file 1364, Morrin to Provincial Secretary, 28 June 1852; Medical Certificate of James Douglas, 28 June 1852; Morrin to Provincial Secretary, 6 July 1852

60 See for example NA, RG4 CI, file 1278, Medical Certificate of Charles Frémont, 30 June 1853; RG4 CI, file 1412, Charles Frémont to Provincial Secretary, 15 July 1853; RG4 CI, file 1270, 1852; RG4 CI, file 2304, Frémont to Provincial Secretary, 22 December 1853

61 NA, RG4 CI, file 2315, Medical Certificate of Charles Frémont, 2 December 1853. Other cases in which proprietors petition for less-than-hopeful cases include: NA, RG4 CI, file 2348, 1856; RG4 CI, file 815, 1854; RG4 CI, file 1547, 1853; RG4 CI, file 1476, 1853.

62 See for example NA, RG4 CI, file 1737, 1853; RG4 CI, file 771, 1853.

63 See for example NA, RG4 CI, file 1706, 1855, where Frémont refers to a patient as "un pauvre diable." See also NA, RG4 CI, file 1475, 1853, for a petition endorsed by Morrin and Frémont concerning a patient whose insanity was said to be of five years' duration without lucid intervals.

64 "La porteuse est la mère d'une jeune fille épileptique et devenue aliénée par désorganisation du cerveau. La pauvre femme est véritablement respectable et mérite d'être secourue. Elle a supporté cette jeune fille depuis bien des années au moyen de ce que lui prouvuroient des soins de garde-malade, mais les choses sont tellement empirées chez elle que la mère et la fille sont menacées de misère ... je n'hésite pas de vous la recommander [pour admission] instamment" NA, RG4 CI, file 1749, Frémont to Provincial Secretary.

65 NA, RG4 CI, file 963, A. Morin to Provincial Secretary, 19 June 1854; Petition of Pierre Leclaire and his wife, 14 June 1854; Provincial Secretary to Leclaire, 19 July 1854; A. Morin to Provincial Secretary, 12 August 1854; Provincial Secretary to Commissioners of the Beauport Lunatic Asylum, 12 August 1854. Similar petitions endorsed by high-ranking political and religious figures invariably received the sanction of the state. See for example NA, RG4 CI, file 148, Bishop of Quebec to Provincial Secretary, 23 January 1857; RG4 CI, file 1371, George Etienne Cartier to Provincial Secretary, 27 April 1848; RG4 CI, file 2857, Dr Joseph Painchaud to Provincial Secretary, December 1852; RG4 CI, file 2030, Wolfred Nelson to Provincial Secretary, 19 June 1849.

66 See Rosenberg, *The Care of Strangers*, 24–5. A similar argument can be found in Vogel, *The Invention of the Modern Hospital*, 1–28.

67 Joseph Morrin and Charles Frémont were instrumental in founding the

faculty of medicine at the University of Laval. James Douglas was visiting physician and chief surgeon to the Quebec Marine and Emigrant Hospital. Biographies of these physicians can be found in Boissonnault, "Joseph Morrin," *Dictionary of Canadian Biography* (hereafter DCB), vol. 9, 572–3; Boissonnault, "Charles-Jacques Frémont," DCB, vol. 9, 286–7; Roy, *La Famille Frémont*, 29–35; Leblond, "James Douglas," DCB, vol. 11, 270–1; James Douglas Jr. Ed., *Journals and Reminiscences of James Douglas, MD.*

68 Biographical detail on Bolduc is found in Kowrach, ed., *Mission of the Columbia.*

69 "Vous n'avez besoin de notifier personne si vous aurez la complaisance de m'accorder mes demandes." NA, RG4 C1, file 1856, Bolduc to Provincial Secretary, 16 June 1856. In another case, Bolduc noted to the government, "Il n'est pas nécessaire de notifier les personnes pour lesquelles je vous fais demandes ci-dessus." NA, RG4 C1, file 279, Bolduc to Provincial Secretary, 19 February 1857

70 Most of the petitions in which Bolduc participated read: "Admission ordered and sent to Rev'd Mr. Bolduc." Crossed out of the form letter granting committal was the sentence: "I enclose the information required for the guidance of the Medical Officers." The reason for this deletion was that Bolduc himself provided the information, presumably on the basis of his correspondence with, and visits to, the patient and others. In several petitions, Bolduc assured the government that "Les informations sur son compte seront fournies avec médicins de l'asile par moi même."

71 NA, RG4 C1, file 2810, Bolduc to Provincial Secretary, 20 November 1856; Bolduc to Provincial Secretary, 1 December 1856; Provincial Secretary to Bolduc, 4 December 1856; Provincial Secretary to Secretary to the Commissioners of the Beauport Lunatic Asylum, 4 December 1856. For other examples of Bolduc's successful transfers between Beauport and the Quebec General Hospital, see NA, RG4 C1, file 798, 1859; RG4 C1, file 553, 1859.

72 NA, RG4 C1, file 1505, Bolduc to Provincial Secretary, 24 June 1859; Medical Certificate of Frémont and Morrin, 6 June 1859; Copy of a report of a Committee of the Executive Council, 11 July 1859

73 "Le nombre des patients est tombé de 382 à 372 et la visite des commissaires à la fin de ce mois va sans doute le faire diminuer encore de 8 à 10. Il y aura de la place pour toutes mes demandes dans le cours de cette année, c'est chose certain." NA, RG4 C1, file 2095, Bolduc to Provincial Secretary, 19 September 1857; "Le secrétaire de la commission de l'asile des aliénés m'a dit ce matin qu'il y avait des fonds nouvellement mis à votre disposition pour l'asile en question. Or, vous n'ignorez pas que cette nouvelle fut pour moi un véritable joie. J'ai des fous et des folles qui n'attendaient que cela. Je vais donc vous faire mes demandes: il y a

de la place pour les recevoir jusqu'au nombre d'environ 400." Provincial
Secretary to Bolduc, 22 September 1857.

74 NA, RG4 C1, file 279, Bolduc to Provincial Secretary, 19 February 1857

75 See for example NA, RG4 C1, file 1320, Bolduc to Provincial Secretary,
11 May 1855.

76 "Si elle ne se montre pas un peu plus traitable je vais être obligé de l'en-
voyer à l'asile sans attendre le retour de ma demande. De sorte que vous
m'obligerez infinisment en dattant son admission de ce jour en cas de
besoin." NA, RG4 C1, file 56, Bolduc to Provincial Secretary, 8 January
1858; Provincial Secretary to Bolduc, 12 January 1858. See also, NA,
RG4 C1, file 3293, Bolduc to Provincial Secretary, 21 December 1855.
See also RG4 C1, file 2985, 1855.

77 NA, RG4 C1, file 787, Bolduc to Provincial Secretary, 26 February 1856

78 NA, RG4 C1, file 2961, Bolduc to Provincial Secretary, 16 November
1858; RG4 C1, file 544, Bolduc to Provincial Secretary, 8 March
1858

79 In one such case, Bolduc informed the government of a "pauvre vieille
des Soeurs de la Charité. Je pense bien qu'elle n'en reviendra pas, mais
aussi, elle ne fera pas long jours." NA, RG4 C1, file 173, Bolduc to
Provincial Secretary, 22 January 1858

80 "Ces deux patients sont des incurables et ... les parents ont l'air de
vouloir se débarrasser d'eux à quelque prise que ce soit. D'après la lettre
qui m'a été écrite, je n'ai pas osé prendre sur moi d'agir comme j'ai déjà
fait pour bon nombre d'autres. J'ai toujours coutume de choisir les
meilleurs cas quand je vous fais des demandes et si je voulais écouter
tous ceux qui me prient de vous écrire, il y aurait maintenant au delà de
600 patients presque tous incurables." NA, RG4 C1, file 1694, Bolduc to
Provincial Secretary, 17 July 1857

81 Bolduc's involvement in the process of patient admissions seems to have
abated by the mid-1860s, a development possibly attributable to his
appointment as procurator of the archdiocese of Quebec. In 1886 he
was given the title "Domestic Prelate" by Pope Leo XIII. He died at
Quebec on 8 May 1889. See Kowrach, ed., *Mission of the Columbia*,
12.

82 AO, RG 22, Lunatic Accounts, Perth County, Joseph Workman to Clerk
of the Peace, 6 March 1858

83 AO, RG 22, Lunatic Accounts, Perth County, Workman to Linton, 7
April 1858

CHAPTER FIVE

1 The Kingston Penitentiary, established in 1835, served Upper and Lower
Canada after the Act of Union in 1840.

2   The concept of "framing" is drawn partly from Rosenberg, "Framing Disease: Illness, Society, and History." See also Porter, "Gout: Framing and Fantasizing Disease." In a similar way, Hacking studies fugue in order to demonstrate "how a psychiatric entity comes into being and then disappears." Hacking, "Les Aliénés Voyageurs"

3   NA, Correspondence of the Provincial Secretary, RG5 C1, file 2222, Draper to Provincial Secretary, 16 December 1841

4   Verdun-Jones and Smandych also include as criminally insane in nineteenth-century Canada, those who "were labelled 'dangerously insane' and subjected to preventive detention." Verdun-Jones and Smandych, "Catch-22 in the Nineteenth Century," 86

5   See for example the case of John Long, NA, RG5 C1, file 527, Mayor of the City of Toronto to Provincial Secretary, 28 April 1837; and the case of Patrick Donolly, Gaol Report (Niagara District) JLAUC, Appendix 44, 1836.

6   See for example the case of Mathew Hynds who was removed from the Wellington District Jail to the Toronto Temporary Lunatic Asylum, NA, RG5 C1, file 2517, 3 January 1842; AO, RG10–20–B–1 Appendix II, General Register and Admission Orders and Histories, 1842. On the transfer of Sophia Baker from the Home District Jail to the Toronto Temporary Lunatic Asylum see, NA, RG5 C1, file 2222, Mr Justice Jones to Provincial Secretary, 11 December 1841; Certificate of Sanity of William Rees, 28 December 1841.

7   This circuitous route from crime to diagnosis to asylum treatment can be traced in the case of Alexander Cameron. Cameron was committed to the Bathurst District Gaol for assault and battery on 12 April 1842. He remained in the local jail until the fall assizes could try his case five months later in September. Owing to Cameron's obvious manifestations of insanity, the grand jury decided not to proceed with a trial in his case. He was still in jail on 3 October when the warden of the Bathurst jail strongly urged that Cameron be delivered to the temporary asylum at Toronto to "undergo medical treatment." In the opinion of the warden, "the temporary prison at Perth [was] very limited in its accommodation and humanity requires that [this] unhappy person should not be indefinitely confined therein under the circumstances of [his] afflicted condition." NA, RG5 C1, file 4499, Petition for Committal of the Grand Jury of Bathurst District, 3 October 1842

8   See JLAUC, Surgeon's Report, Provincial Penitentiary, 31 December 1853. With the Act of Union in 1841, legislation was passed to "render the Penitentiary erected near Kingston in the Midland District, the Provincial Penitentiary for Canada." Splane notes that although "Canada East did, after a few months, begin to commit prisoners in considerable numbers [to the penitentiary], Upper Canada always provided a dispropor-

tionate percentage of the inmates." Splane, *Social Welfare in Ontario*, 136. Not surprisingly, Sampson also treated more criminal lunatics from Canada West than from the eastern province.

9 *JLAUC*, Surgeon's Report, Kingston Penitentiary, 1850

10 See Sampson's "Return of Insane Convicts," *JLAUC*, Appendix "III", 1 October 1851.

11 *JLAUC*, Appendix "III", Report of the Inspectors of the Provincial Penitentiary, 1852

12 *JLAUC*, Appendix "DD", Surgeon's Report, 31 December 1853

13 Quotations from Splane, *Social Welfare in Ontario*, 138–9

14 See *JLAUC*, Appendix B.B.B.B., 1849, for cases of five insane prisoners aggravated by excessive punishment.

15 The 1848–1849 Royal Commission had originally proposed the creation of a criminal lunatic asylum connected to the penitentiary. The opening of the Toronto Asylum in 1850 may have made the transfer of criminal lunatics to that institution appear to be an easier and cheaper alternative. Section 46 of the Penitentiary Act stated: "Whenever it shall be certified by a Board of Physicians ... that any convict confined therein is insane, and that it is desirable that such convict should be removed therefrom to the Lunatic Asylum, it shall be lawful for the Governor by Warrant under his hand directed to the Warden of said Penitentiary to authorize him forthwith to send such convict to the Lunatic Asylum of Upper Canada." (14–15 Vict., Ch. 2.)

16 This Board was made up of James Sampson, Thomas W. Robinson MD, and John R. Dickson MD. See NA, RG5 C1, file 1836, 1851.

17 *JLAUC*, Surgeon's Report, 1852

18 See 14–15 Vict., Ch. 83. As we shall see, this more general section of the act was to be the source of considerable confusion and conflict later in the century.

19 *JLAUC*, Superintendent's Annual Report, 1852

20 *JLAUC*, Superintendent's Annual Report, 1854, (Emphasis added.)

21 Ibid. See also Oliver, '*Terror to Evil-Doers*', 232

22 See for instance the case of John Osterhout, who was convicted for stealing a skiff in an effort to "cross over to the United States," NA, RG5 C1, 1853, file 1794.

23 These patients are discussed in NA, RG5 C1, file 585, 1854. Workman eventually pronounced them both cured.

24 NA, RG5 C1, file 1492, Report of the Medical Superintendent, 20 September 1853

25 *JLAUC*, Surgeon's Report, 1853

26 *JLAUC*, Surgeon's Report, 31 December 1853. Although their transfer was not legally sanctioned at the official level, it is clear that in some cases criminals from Quebec who ended up at the Kingston Penitentiary

and who were subsequently found to be insane were rerouted to the Beauport Asylum. In one case, a French Canadian prisoner at the Kingston Penitentiary who had become insane was ordered by law to be transferred to the Toronto Asylum. But before she was sent, the Provincial Secretary intervened and changed her institutional destination to the Beauport Asylum. See NA, RG4 C1, file 2189, Warden of the Kingston Penitentiary to Provincial Secretary, 29 July 1856.

27   NA, RG4 C1, file 14, The Queen *vs* Anne Dupont – Indictment for Infanticide, March 1853; The Queen *vs* Anne Dupont, 17 March 1853; Report of Morrin and Frémont on the Mental State of Anne Dupont, 20 December 1854; Provincial Secretary to Beauport Proprietors, 5 January 1855. RG4 C1, file 527, Marchand to Provincial Secretary, 7 April 1854; Provincial Secretary to Marchand, 12 April 1854; Report of the Attorney General on the Case of Marchand, 11 April 1856. See also RG4 C1, 14, Attorney General to Beauport Proprietors, 5 January 1855.

28   See for example Macdonald to Provincial Secretary, 1 December 1854, "In the matter of James McDonell an inmate of the Provincial Lunatic Asylum"; Macdonald to Provincial Secretary, January 1855, "The convict Needham ... convicted on two indictments for larceny & acquitted on the third on the ground of insanity," in Johnson, ed., *The Letters of Sir John A. Macdonald*, 218–19; 222.

29   See Angus, "James Sampson"; Travill, *Medicine at Queen's*, 6; Angus, "John Dickson."

30   Macdonald's report was acted upon in a Report of a Committee of the Executive Council, 2 March 1855. The Executive Committee also endorsed "a permanent asylum for the criminal insane [to] be erected in the penitentiary farm" and "a bill [to] be introduced during the present session to authorise the employment of convicts under certain regulations, beyond the walls to assist in the construction of the building referred to." See NA, RG5 C1, file 194, Macdonald to Provincial Secretary, 27 February 1855; and Report of the Executive Council, 2 March 1855.

31   Macdonald to Provincial Secretary, 5 March 1855, in Johnson, *Letters*, 251–2

32   Litchfield's journalistic pursuits put him into contact with several members of Upper Canada's medical and political elite who saw in him a logical solution to some of their pressing concerns. Litchfield served for a short period in 1854 as editor of the *Montreal Pilot*, a Reform Party newspaper. The social and political connections generated through his position as editor led to his appointment in March 1855 as head of the Montreal committee for choosing Canadian exhibits for the upcoming Paris International Exhibition. This appointment offered Litchfield further opportunity to socialize with prominent members of the Canadian

political elite at a committee luncheon, attended by the new Governor General, Sir Edmond Bond Head, and the mayor of Montreal. See Gibson, "The Astonishing Career of John Palmer Litchfield."

33   Litchfield was subsequently appointed on 20 June to the first official medical faculty at Queen's University as professor of midwifery and state and forensic medicine. In his lectures on medical jurisprudence, he would work with Alexander Campbell, the law partner of John A. Macdonald. There is some dispute about whether Litchfield was in fact a licensed practitioner. His "questionable" background is the focus of much of Gibson's unpublished paper "The Astonishing Career of John Palmer Litchfield." However, there is ample evidence of his medical credentials, (including copies of his medical licence, a 5 year superintendency at the private Walton Asylum in England, and physician's referrals) in the records of the Provincial Secretary. See NA RG5 CI, file 176.

34   Workman considered this decision and the consequent removal of all criminally insane patients as "a blessing to the [Toronto Asylum], the true value of which can be appreciated only by those who were cognizant of the evil caused by their presence here." *JLAUC*, Superintendent's Annual Report, 1856. Sampson also appeared pleased to see "a separate establishment lately formed for the management and safe keeping of that unfortunate class of individuals." *JLAUC*, Surgeon's Report, 1855

35   *JLAUC*, Report of Wolfred Nelson and Andrew Dickson, 1857

36   Litchfield's position as superintendent of the Walton Lunatic Asylum is documented in NA, RG4 CI, file 2473.

37   See for example Litchfield's Annual Report for 1866, *JLAUC*.

38   A description of the new Rockwood Criminal Lunatic Asylum can be found in Henry Hurd, ed., *Institutional Care of the Insane*, 149. See also the descriptions by the asylum's architect, William Cloverdale, in *JLAUC*, Architect's Report, 1861, and by Litchfield in *JLAUC*, Annual Report, 1861.

39   Hurd, *Institutional Care of the Insane*, 148. Surgeon Sampson made clear his objections to this accommodation for female patients in the following satirical verse:

> O would to God that I were able
> To build a house like Cartwright's stable.
> For it would fill me with remorse
> To be worse housed than Cartwright's horse.

See Gibson, "The Astonishing Career of John Palmer Litchfield."

40   NA, RG5 CI, file 865, copy of a Report of a Committee of the Honourable Provincial Secretary, approved 12 July 1856; also file 487, Litchfield to Provincial Secretary, 25 March 1857. Litchfield also secured space in the dwelling house of the estate to set up a private asylum. Fees

from private patients were meant to offset some of the public expense incurred in treating other criminal lunatics. NA, RG5 C1, file 772, Litchfield to Provincial Secretary, 2 May 1857; file 1147 Litchfield to Provincial Secretary, 24 June 1857; see also file 1497, copy of a Licence Authorising Litchfield to Keep a Private Asylum. In 1861, three years before the opening of the new Rockwood Asylum, more asylum provision was provided with the purchase of the Cartwright Cottage at Rockwood. NA, RG4 C1, file 378, Report of a Committee of the Executive Council Approved by His Excellency the Governor General in Council, 21 September 1861

41 NA, RG5 C1, file 768, Litchfield to Provincial Secretary, 12 May 1855
42 See *JLAUC*, General Inspectors' Report, 1860; *JLAUC*, Report of Inspector Wolfred Nelson, 1860; *JLAUC*, Report of Inspector Terrence O'Neill, 1864
43 As early as 1858 the warden of the penitentiary complained: "The space they [criminal lunatics] now occupy is much required for storage of provisions for the use of the convicts," *JLAUC*, Annual Report of the Provincial Penitentiary, 1858.
44 *JLAUC*, Litchfield's Annual Report, 1861. In 1857 there were twenty-four male patients in the basement asylum. By 1858 the number had reached fifty-nine. By 1862 there were sixty-four patients and in 1864 the total was seventy-two. Respective figures for female patients in the "stable-asylum" and the Rockwood estate were fifteen, twenty-six, twenty-three, and twenty-six.
45 *JLAUC*, General Inspectors' Report, 1865
46 *JLAUC*, Litchfield's Annual Report, 1859
47 *JLAUC*, See for example Litchfield's Annual Report, 1860.
48 *JLAUC*, Litchfield's Annual Report, 1862
49 *JLAUC*, See Litchfield's Annual Report, 1863, and General Report of the Inspectors, 1864.
50 *JLAUC*, Litchfield's Annual Reports, 1863 and 1865
51 To this end Litchfield created thirty small single dormitories in the penitentiary basement and a "sick bay" with associated dormitory with space for twenty patients. The total capacity of this arrangement was approximately fifty patients, and it was perhaps an indication of the health problems manifested in the asylum that two-fifths of the organized space was designed for those who were sick and convalescent. This arrangement became increasingly cramped with the growth of the male patient population, and by 1860 Litchfield was forced to build sleeping bunks in the corridors along the sides of the dormitories. *JLAUC*, Report of Dr Wolfred Nelson, 1861; *JLAUC*, Litchfield's Annual Report, 1860. Oliver also discusses conditions in this temporary asylum in '*Terror to Evil-Doers*', 234–6.

52 *JLAUC*, See Litchfield's Annual Report, 1866.

53 NA, RG4 B65, file 1193; AO, Litchfield's Directory of Patients, Patient No. 190

54 Case of Robert Davis, NA, RG5 C1, file 1084, Petition for the Release of Robert Davis, 21 February 1860; Litchfield to Provincial Secretary, 21 August 1860, and 3 October 1860. See also Case of William Henry Nelson, NA, RG5 C1, file 535.

55 NA, RG5 C1, file 1437, Memorial of Johathan Cloverdale, 10 December 1864; Litchfield to Provincial Secretary, 24 December 1864; Litchfield to Provincial Secretary, 18 April 1864. For another example of this kind of probationary release strategy see Case of Robert Davis, NA, RG5 C1, file 1084; and Case of Thomas Kearn, NA, RG5 C1, file 1624.

56 Case of James Jackson, *JLAUC*, Report of the Rockwood Criminal Lunatic Asylum for 1866; AO, Litchfield's Directory of Patients, Patient No. 22. See also the case of Charles Heybourne, in *JLAUC*, Report of the Rockwood Criminal Lunatic Asylum for 1866; AO, Litchfield's Directory of Patients, Patient No. 231.

57 *JLAUC*, Litchfield's Annual Report, 1866

58 NA, RG5 C1, file 1178, Report of Wolfred Nelson to Provincial Secretary, 18 August 1859

59 Ibid.

60 Ibid.

61 Workman did, however, concur with the prison inspector about certain practical amendments to the plans for the new institution.

62 NA, RG5 C1, file 1178, Joseph Workman to Provincial Secretary, 18 August 1859

63 Ibid.

64 *JLAUC*, Report of Inspectors Nelson and Dickson, 1856

65 See NA, RG5 C1, file 1076, Provincial Secretary to John Litchfield, 26 July 1855.

66 See *JLAUC*, Litchfield's Annual Reports, 1866 and 1864; *JLAUC*, Inspectors' Report, 1864.

67 Litchfield's Annual Report, 1866, *JLAUC*

68 *JLAUC*, Dickson's Annual Report, 1872

69 This transfer coincided with the purchase of the Rockwood Asylum from the Federal Government by the Province of Ontario. See *An Act Respecting the Transfer of Rockwood Asylum to the Province of Ontario, and to Amend the Penitentiary Act of 1875*, 40 Vict., Ch. 38, 1877.

70 Tuke, *The Insane in the United States and Canada*, 237–8

71 Ibid.

72 See *Report of the Royal Commission on Penitentiaries*, 1914.

CONCLUSION

1   Katz, Doucet and Stern discuss the "birth of the institutional state," comprising "mental hospitals, schools systems, reformatories, and penitentiaries" in, *The Social Organization of Early Industrial Capitalism,* 349–91. See also the collection of essays in Greer and Radforth eds., *Colonial Leviathan.*

2   Curtis, *Building the Educational State;* Curtis, *True Government by Choice Men?*

3   Curtis, *True Government,* 5–6

4   Ibid. 11. Susan Houston and Alison Prentice have their own analysis of the development of the state and education which, while sharing common ground with Curtis, is different in several respects. Houston and Prentice, *Schooling and Scholars in Nineteenth-Century Ontario.*

5   Although success of this asylum agenda has been the subject of much scholarly debate in recent years, the agenda itself is clearly elaborated in countless annual reports and propaganda tracts of nineteenth-century asylum advocates. Some of this material is well synthesized in Rothman's, *The Discovery of the Asylum,* 137–54. A detailed discussion of the importance of architecture in the regulation of madness can be found in Tomes, *A Generous Confidence,* 129–88.

6   Scull argues that "moral treatment actively sought to *transform* the lunatic, to remodel him into something approximating the bourgeois ideal of the rational individual." Scull, "Moral Treatment Reconsidered," 89. This theme is emphasized in Michel Foucault, *Madness and Civilization,* 178–241.

7   The symbolic and practical incorporation of science into nineteenth-century medical practice is discussed in Bynum, *Science and the Practice of Medicine.* For an account of physicians' use of "not the content, but the rhetoric of science" in their pursuit of professional and socioeconomic status in the nineteenth century, see Shortt, "Physicians, Science and Status." The "medical capture of madness" in nineteenth-century English psychiatry is discussed in Scull, *The Most Solitary of Afflictions,* 3–4. Elsewhere I have argued that mid-century American alienists used the rhetoric of professional and medical authority in an effort to supplant entrenched customs of community care of the insane with asylum care. See Moran, "Asylum in the Community." Goldstein discusses the struggle of the French psychiatric profession to secularize and medicalize the care of the insane in *Console and Classify.*

8   Scull, *The Most Solitary of Afflictions,* 30

9   See Grob, *The State and the Mentally Ill;* Grob, *Mental Institutions in America*

10 Baehre, "Imperial Authority and Colonial Officialdom of Upper Canada in the 1830s"
11 See Fecteau, *Un nouvel ordre des choses*; Katz, *The Social Organization of Early Industrial Capitalism*, Ch. 9
12 Little, *State and Society in Transition*, 240
13 Curtis, *Building the Educational State*, 373

Bibliography

PRIMARY SOURCES

Archival Collections

National Archives of Canada, Ottawa
Correspondence of the Provincial Secretary, Canada East
  Superintendents' Reports
  Jail Surgeons' Reports and Correspondence
  Jail Wardens' Reports and Correspondence
  Clerk of the Peace Reports and Correspondence
  Provincial Secretary's Reports
  Reports of the Executive Council
  Petitions for Asylum Committal and Correspondence
  Medical Certificates of Insanity
  General Correspondence on Asylum Affairs
Correspondence of the Provincial Secretary, Canada West
  Superintendents' Reports
  Jail Surgeons' Reports and Correspondence
  Jail Wardens' Reports and Correspondence
  Clerk of the Peace Reports and Correspondence
  Provincial Secretary's Reports
  Reports of the Executive Council
  Petitions for Asylum Committal and Correspondence
  Medical Certificates of Insanity
  General Correspondence on Asylum Affairs

Archives of Ontario, Toronto

Ontario Sessional Papers
Correspondence of the Inspector of Prisons and Private Charities
Journals of the Legislative Assembly of Upper Canada
Clerk of the Peace, Lunatic Accounts, Perth County, Unprocessed Correspondence
Statutes of Upper Canada

Archives nationales, Québec

Quebec Sessional Papers
Journals of the Legislative House of Lower Canada

Published Sources

Annual Report of the Medical Superintendent of the Temporary Provincial Lunatic Asylum, At Toronto. Toronto: Scobie and Balfour, 1847
Canada Medical Journal and Monthly Record of Medical and Surgical Science, 1853–57.
Park, George. *A Narrative of the Recent Difficulties in the Provincial Lunatic Asylum in Canada West.* Toronto: Toronto Examiner, 1849
Prichard, J.C. *A Treatise on Insanity and Other Disorders Affecting the Mind.* London: Sherwood, Gilbert, and Piper, 1835
Report of the Royal Commission on Lunatic Asylums of the Province of Quebec. Quebec, 1888
Report of the Royal Commission on Penitentiaries. Ottawa, 1914
Rush, Benjamin. *Medical Inquiries and Observations Upon the Diseases of the Mind.* Philadelphia: Kimber and Richardson, 1818
Rules and Regulations of the Montreal Lunatic Asylum for the Government of the Officers, Patients and Servants of the Institution. Montreal: James Starke and Co., 1840

SECONDARY SOURCES

Alexander, Franz and S. Selesnick. *The History of Psychiatry*: An Evaluation of Psychiatric Thought and Practice from Prehistoric Times to the Present. New York: Harper and Row, 1966
Angus, Margaret. "James Sampson," *Dictionary of Canadian Biography* (hereafter DCB), vol. 9, 699–701. Toronto: University of Toronto Press, 1976
– "John Dickson," DCB, vol. 10 (1977), 268
Baehre, Rainer. *The Ill-Regulated Mind: A Study in the Making of Psychiatry in Ontario, 1830–1921.* PhD thesis, Department of History, York University, 1985

- "Imperial Authority and Colonial Officialdom of Upper Canada in the 1830s: The State, Crime, Lunacy and Everyday Social Order," in Louis Knafla and Susan Binnie eds. *Law, Society and the State: Essays in Modern Legal History.* Toronto: University of Toronto Press, 1995, 181–214

Bartlett, Peter and David Wright eds.. *Outside the Walls of the Asylum: The History of Care in the Community, 1750-2000.* London: Athlone Press, 1999

Boissonnault, Charles-Marie. "Joseph Morrin," DCB, vol. 9, 572–3

- "Charles-Jacques Frémont," DCB, vol. 9, 286–7

Bradbury, Bettina. *Working Families: Age, Gender and Daily Survival in Industrializing Montreal.* Toronto: McClelland & Stewart, 1993

Brown, Thomas E. *"Living with God's Afflicted": A History of the Provincial Lunatic Asylum at Toronto, 1830–1911.* PhD Thesis, Department of History, Kingston University, 1980

- "Dance of the Dialectic? Some Reflections (Academic and Otherwise) on the Recent State of Nineteenth-Century Asylum Studies," *Canadian Bulletin of Medical History,* 11 (1994), 267–95

- "Architecture as Therapy," *Archivaria* 10 (1980), 109–117

Burgess, T.J.W. "A Historical Sketch of Our Canadian Institutions for the Insane," *Transactions of the Royal Society of Canada* 4 (1898), 3–122

Bynum, W.F. *Science and the Practice of Medicine in the Nineteenth Century.* Cambridge: Cambridge University Press, 1994

- "Nosology," in *Companion Encyclopedia to the History of Medicine.* London: Routledge, 1993

Castel, Robert. *The Regulation of Madness: The Origins of Incarceration in France.* Cambridge: Polity Press, 1988

Cellard, André. *Histoire de la folie au Québec, de 1600 à 1850: le désordre.* Québec: Boréal, 1991

Cellard, André and D. Nadon, "Ordre et désordre: le Montreal Lunatic Asylum et la naissance de l'asile au Québec," *Revue d'histoire de l'Amérique française* 39 (Winter, 1986), 345–69

Connor, James T. "'A Sort of Felo-De-Se': Eclecticism, Related Medical Sects and Their Decline in Victorian Ontario," *Bulletin of the History of Medicine* 65 (1991), 503–27

Curtis, Bruce. *Building the Educational State: Canada West, 1836–1871.* London: The Althouse Press, 1988

- *True Government by Choice Men? Inspection, Education and State Formation in Canada West.* Toronto: University of Toronto Press, 1992

Digby, Ann. *Madness, Morality and Medicine: A Study of the York Retreat, 1796–1914.* Cambridge: Cambridge University Press, 1985

Doerner, Klaus. *Madmen and the Bourgeoisie: A Social History of Insanity and Psychiatry.* Oxford: Basil Blackwell, 1986

Douglas, James, Jr. *Journals and Reminiscences of James Douglas, M.D.* New York: Torch Press, 1910

Dowbiggin, Ian. *Keeping America Sane: Psychiatry and Eugenics in the United States and Canada, 1880–1940*. Ithica: Cornell University Press, 1997

Duffin, Jacalyn. *Langstaff: A Nineteenth-Century Medical Life*. Toronto: University of Toronto Press, 1993

Dwyer, Ellen. *Homes for the Mad: Life Inside Two Nineteenth-Century Asylums*. New Brunswick: Rutgers University Press, 1987

Fecteau, Jean-Marie. *Un nouvel ordre des choses: La pauvreté, le crime, l'état au Québec de la fin du XVIII siècle à 1840*. Québec: VLB éditeur, 1989

Finnane, Mark. "Asylums, Families and the State," *History Workshop Journal* 20 (1985)

– *Insanity and the Insane in Post-Famine Ireland*. London: Croom Helm, 1981

Foucault, Michel. *Déraison et folie: histoire de la folie à l'âge classique*. Paris: Plon, 1961

– *Madness and Civilization: A History of Insanity in the Age of Reason*. New York: Random House, 1965

Gibson, Thomas. "The Astonishing Career of John Palmer Litchfield, First Professor of Forensic Medicine at Queen's University, Kingston," unpublished manuscript

Gidney, R.D., and W. Miller. "Origins of Organized Medicine in Ontario," in *Health, Disease and Medicine: Essays in Canadian History*. Toronto: Hannah Institute for the History of Medicine, 1984, 65–95

Goldstein, Jan. *Console and Classify: The French Psychiatric Profession in the Nineteenth Century*. Cambridge: Cambridge University Press, 1987

– "'The Lively Sensibility of the Frenchman': Some Reflections on the Place of France in Foucault's *Histoire de la folie*," *History of the Human Sciences* 3 (1990), 3–26

Greer, Allen, and Ian Radforth eds. *Colonial Leviathan: State Formation in Mid-Nineteenth-Century Canada*. Toronto: University of Toronto Press, 1992

Grob, Gerald. *The State and the Mentally Ill: A History of Worcester State Hospital in Massachusetts, 1830–1920*. Chapel Hill: University of North Carolina Press, 1965

– *Mental Institutions in America: Social Policy to 1875*. New York: The Free Press, 1973

– *Mental Illness and American Society, 1875–1914*. Princeton: Princeton University Press, 1983

– *From Asylum to Community: Mental Health Policy in Modern America*. Princeton: Princeton University Press, 1994

– "Marxian Analysis and Mental Illness," *History of Psychiatry* 1 (1990), 223–32

– *The Mad Among Us: A History of the Care of America's Mentally Ill*. New York: The Free Press, 1994

Hacking, Ian. "Les Aliénés Voyageurs: How Fugue Became a Medical Entity," *History of Psychiatry* 7 (1996), 425–49

Hannaway, Caroline. "Environment and Miasmata," in W.F. Bynum and R. Porter eds. *Companion Encyclopedia of the History of Medicine.* London: Routledge, 1993, 293–308

Houston, Susan, and Alison Prentice. *Schooling and Scholars in Nineteenth-Century Ontario.* Toronto: University of Toronto Press, 1988

Hurd, Henry, ed. *The Institutional Care of the Insane in the United States and Canada.* Baltimore: Johns Hopkins University Press, 1916

Jiminez, Mary Ann. *Changing Faces of Madness: Early American Attitudes and Treatment of the Insane.* Hanover: University Press of New England, 1987

Johnson, J.K., ed. *The Letters of Sir John A. Macdonald, 1836-1857.* vol. 1, Ottawa: Public Archives, 1968

Katz, Michael, Michael Doucet, and Mark Stern. *The Social Organization of Early Industrial Capitalism.* Cambridge: Harvard University Press, 1982

Keating, Peter. *La science du mal: L'institution de la psychiatrie au Québec, 1800–1914.* Québec: Boréal, 1993

Kowrach, Edward J. ed. *Mission of the Columbia: Jean Baptiste Zacharie Bolduc.* Washington: Ye Galleon Press, 1979

Leblond, Sylvio. "James Douglas," DCB, vol. 2 (1982), 270–1

Little, J.I. *State and Society in Transition: The Politics of Institutional Reform in the Eastern Townships, 1838-1852.* Kingston: McGill-Queen's University Press, 1997

McCandless, Peter. *Moonlight, Magnolias and Madness: Insanity in North Carolina from the Colonial Period to the Progressive Era.* Chapel Hill: University of North Carolina Press, 1996

Middlefort, H.C.E. "Madness and Civilization in Early Modern Europe," in *After the Reformation: Essays in Honor of J.H. Hexer.* Philadelphia: University of Pennsylvania Press, 1980

Mitchinson, Wendy. *The Nature of their Bodies: Women and their Doctors in Victorian Canada.* Toronto: University of Toronto Press, 1991

– "Reasons for Committal to a Mid-Nineteenth-Century Ontario Insane Asylum: The Case of Toronto," in Mitchinson, Wendy and Janice Dickin McGinnis, eds., *Essays in the History of Canadian Medicine.* Toronto: McClelland & Stewart, 1988, 88–109

Mora, George. "The History of Psychiatry in the United States: Historiographic and Theoretical Considerations," *History of Psychiatry* 1 (1992), 187–201

Moran, James E. "Asylum in the Community: Managing the Insane in Antebellum America," *History of Psychiatry,* 9, (1998), 1–24

– "Keepers of the Insane: The Role of Attendants at the Toronto Provincial Asylum, 1875–1905," *Histoire sociale/Social History* 18 (1995), 51–75

Oliver, Peter. 'Terror to Evil-Doers': Prisons and Punishments in Nineteenth-Century Ontario. Toronto: University of Toronto Press, 1998

Parr, Joy. The Gender of Breadwinners. Toronto: University of Toronto Press, 1990

Perkin, Harold. The Origins of Modern English Society, 1789–1880. London: Routledge and Paul, 1969

Porter, Roy. Mind-Forg'd Manacles: A History of Madness in England from the Restoration to the Regency. London: Athlone, 1987

– "Foucault's Great Confinement," History of the Human Sciences 3 (1990), 47–54.

– "Madness and its Institutions," in Wear, Andrew, ed. Medicine in Modern Society: Historical Essays. Cambridge: Cambridge University Press, 1992

– "Gout: Framing and Fantasizing Disease," Bulletin of the History of Medicine 68 (1994), 1–28

Prestwich, Patricia E.. "Family Strategies and Medical Power: 'Voluntary' Committal in a Parisian Asylum, 1876–1914," Journal of Social History 27 (1994), 799–818

Reaume, Geoffrey. 999 Queen Street West: Patient Life at the Toronto Hospital for the Insane, 1870–1940. PhD Thesis, Department of History, University of Toronto, 1997

Ripa, Yannick. Women and Madness: The Incarceration of Women in Nineteenth-Century France. Minneapolis: University of Minneapolis Press, 1990

Rosenberg, Charles. The Care of Strangers: The Rise of America's Hospital System. Baltimore: Johns Hopkins University Press, 1987

– "Framing Disease: Illness, Society, and History," in Rosenberg, Charles, and Janet Olden eds. Framing Disease: Studies in Cultural History. New Brunswick: Rutgers University Press, 1992

Rothman, David. The Discovery of the Asylum: Social Order and Disorder in the New Republic. Boston: Little Brown, 1971

Roy, Pierre Georges. La famille Frémont. Lévis, 1902

Scull, Andrew. Social Order/Mental Disorder: Anglo-American Psychiatry in Historical Perspective. Berkeley: University of California Press, 1989

– Museums of Madness: The Social Organization of Insanity in Nineteenth-Century England. London: Allen Lane, 1979

– "Michel Foucault's History of Madness," History of the Human Sciences 3 (1990), 57–67

– "A Failure to Communicate? On the Reception of Foucault's Histoire de la folie by Anglo-American Historians," in Still, Arthur and Irving Velody eds. Rewriting the History of Madness: Studies in Foucault's Histoire de la folie. London: Routledge, 1992, 150–63

– The Most Solitary of Afflictions: Madness and Society in Britain, 1700–1900. New Haven: Yale University Press, 1993

- "Mental Health Policy in Modern America," *The Millbank Quarterly* 70 (1992)
- "Psychiatry and Social Control in the Nineteenth and Twentieth Centuries," *History of Psychiatry* 2 (1991), 239–50
- "Reflections on the Historical Sociology of Psychiatry," in Scull, ed. *Social Order/Mental Disorder: Anglo-American Psychiatry in Historical Perspective*. Berkeley: University of California Press, 1989

Shorter, Edward. *A History of Psychiatry: From the Era of the Asylum to the Age of Prozac*. New York: John Wiley and Sons, 1997

Shortt, S.E.D. "Physicians, Science and Status: Issues in the Professionalization of Anglo-American Medicine in the Nineteenth Century," *Medical History* 27 (1983), 51–68 *Victorian Lunacy: Richard M. Bucke and the Practice of Late Nineteenth-Century Psychiatry*. Cambridge: Cambridge University Press, 1986
- *Victorian Lunacy: Richard M. Bucke and the Practice of Late Nineteenth-Century Psychiatry*. Cambridge: Cambridge University Press, 1986

Showalter, Elaine. *The Female Malady: Women, Madness and English Culture, 1830–1980*. New York: Pantheon, 1985

Splane, Richard. *Social Welfare in Ontario, 1791–1893*. Toronto: University of Toronto Press, 1965

Stalwick, H. *A History of Asylum Administration in Pre-Confederation Canada*. PhD thesis, University of London, 1969

Stevenson, Christine. "Medicine and Architecture," in W.F. Bynum and Roy Porter eds. *Companion Encyclopedia of the History of Medicine*. London: Routledge, 1993, 293–308

Stone, Lawrence. *The Past and the Present Revisited*. London: Routledge and Kegan Paul, 1987

Thompson, E.P.T. *The Making of the English Working Class*. London: Penguin Books, 1968

Travill, A.A. *Medicine at Queen's: A Particularly Happy Relationship*. Kingston: McGill-Queen's University Press, 1988

Tomes, Nancy. "The Anatomy of Madness: New Directions in the History of Psychiatry," *Social Studies of Science* 17 (1987)
- *A Generous Confidence: Thomas Story Kirkbride and the Art of Asylum-Keeping, 1840–1883*. Cambridge: Cambridge University Press, 1984

Travill, A.A. *Medicine at Queen's: A Particularly Happy Relationship*. Kingston: McGill-Queen's University Press, 1988

Tuke, Daniel Hacke. *The Insane in the United States and Canada*. London: Lewis, 1885

Verdun-Jones, Simon, and Russell Smandych. "Catch-22 in the Nineteenth Century: The Evolution of Therapeutic Confinement for the Criminally Insane in Canada, 1840–1900," *Criminal Justice History* 2 (1981), 85–108

Vogel, Morris J. *The Invention of the Modern Hospital: Boston, 1870–1930*. Chicago: Chicago University Press, 1980

Walton, John. "Casting Out and Bringing Back in Victorian England: Pauper Lunatics, 1840–70," in Bynum, W.F. et al eds. *The Anatomy of Madness*. vol. 2. London: Tavistock, 1985, 132–46

Warsh, Sheryl. *Moments of Unreason: The Practice of Canadian Psychiatry and the Homewood Retreat*. Montreal: McGill-Queen's University Press, 1989

Wright, David. "Getting Out of the Asylum: Understanding Confinement of the Insane in the Nineteenth Century," *Social History of Medicine* 10 (1997), 137–55

Zilboorg, Gregory. *A History of Medical Psychology*. New York: Norton, 1941

Index